INTERMITTENT FASTING FOR WOMEN OVER 50

The Essential Beginners Guide to Lose Weight Rapidly and Burn Fat. Reset Metabolism, Change and Improve your Habits, Increase your Life Energy and Detox your Body by Healthy Recipes

Olivia Keller

Copyright © 2021 Olivia Keller

All rights reserved.

The purpose of this document is to provide accurate and credible information on the subject and problem at hand. The book is sold on the understanding that the publisher is not obligated to provide accounting, legally authorized, or otherwise eligible services. If legal or technical advice is needed, a well-versed professional should be consulted.

A Committee of the American Bar Association and a Committee of Publishers and Associations have adopted and endorsed the Declaration of Principles.

Whether in electronic or written format, any part of this publication must not be reproduced, duplicated, or transmitted in any manner. The recording of this publication is strictly forbidden, and preservation of this text is only permitted with the publisher's written permission. The intellectual property rights are reserved.

The details given herein are claimed to be true and consistent, in that any liability arising from the use or misuse of any rules, procedures, or instructions contained herein, whether due to inattention or otherwise, is solely and completely the responsibility of the receiver reader. In no condition will the publisher be found liable for any reparation, negligence, or monetary injury incurred as a result of the details contained herein, whether directly or indirectly.

The copyrights not owned by the

publisher belong to the authors.

The knowledge included here is strictly for educational purposes and is thus universal. The knowledge is presented without some kind of contract or promise assurance.

The logos are used without the trademark owner's permission or backing, and the trademark is published without the trademark owner's permission or backing. The trademarks and logos mentioned in this book are the property of their respective owners and are not associated with this document.

TABLE OF CONTENTS

INTRODUCTION 14

INTERMITTENT FASTING FOR FAT LOSS: GOOD OR BAD? 22

    Intermittent Fasting 101: 23

    Things to consider during your fast: 24

    Things to consider during your Feeding or Fed state: 25

    Pros and Cons of Intermittent Fasting + General Guidelines: 26

    Guidelines: 26

INTERMITTENT FASTING, ADF, OR 5:2 FASTING IS EFFECTIVE? 28

    Is the 5:2 diet different from intermittent fasting? 28

    Why choose the 5:2 diet? 29

    Does 5:2 diet push your body to starvation mode? 29

    Benefits of 5:2 diet 30

INTERMITTENT FASTING VS LOW CARB DIET? ... 32

    Beneficial Low Carb Intermittent Fasting 35

INTERMITTENT FASTING SCHEDULE 38

    Weekly Intermittent Fasting 41

    Alternate Day Intermittent Fasting 43

    Seven ways to do intermittent fasting 46

1. Fast for 12 hours a day 46

2. Fasting for 16 hours 47

3. Fasting for 2 days a week 48

4. Alternate day fasting 50

5. A weekly 24-hour fast 51

6. Meal skipping 52

7. The Warrior Diet 53

Tips for maintaining intermittent fasting 54

INTERMITTENT FASTING MEAL PLANS 57

Weeks One and Two: The 5:2 Plan 59

Beyond the Fasting Window 62

Next Steps: Will I Stick With IF? 62

1. Water 68

2. Avocado 69

3. Fish and seafood 70

4. Cruciferous veggies 70

5. Potatoes 71

5. Beans and legumes 71

6. Probiotics 72

7. Berries 73

8. Eggs 73

9. Nuts 74

WHAT MAKES INTERMITTENT FASTING WORK? 76

WHAT IS INTERMITTENT FASTING (IF)?............. 76
TYPES OF INTERMITTENT FASTING:................... 79
- 1. ALTERNATE DAY FASTING:........................... 80
- 2. MODIFIED FASTING - 5:2 DIET...................... 80
- 3. TIME-RESTRICTED FEEDING:........................ 82

COMMON QUESTION ABOUT INTERMITTENT FASTING:.. 84
- IF YOU JUST WANT THE BENEFITS:.................. 85
- To recap, here are the possible benefits of intermittent fasting:.. 85

THE FACT THAT FASTING FOR WEIGHT LOSS IS SO SUCCESSFUL HAS TWO MAIN REASONS. 91
- 1. Fat burning will occur if there is little to no food in the body. 91
- 2. Fasting Is A Simple Way To Reduce Calories Without Forgoing The Foods You Enjoy. 91
- My two preferred techniques for fasting are:................... 92

HOW TO LOSE WEIGHT BY INTERMITTENT FASTING? 95

7 REASONS WHY YOU SHOULD CONSIDER INTERMITTENT FASTING - APART FROM WEIGHT LOSS 101
- 1. Intermittent fasting may help maintain muscle. 104
- 2. Intermittent fasting may target belly fat................ 105
- 3. Intermittent fasting may reduce diabetes risk. 106

4. Intermittent fasting may lower high blood pressure. 107

5. Intermittent fasting could fight inflammation. 107

6. Intermittent fasting may reduce oxidative stress. ... 108

7. Intermittent fasting may help you live longer. 109

SIDE EFFECTS OF INTERMITTENT FASTING? 110

Below are two metabolic changes that occur when you fast : 110

4 INTERMITTENT FASTING SIDE EFFECTS TO WATCH OUT FOR 113

The most common forms include: 114

#1. Intermittent fasting may make you feel sick. 115

#2. It may cause you to overeat. 115

#3. Intermittent fasting may cause older adults to lose too much weight. 116

#4. It may be dangerous if you're taking certain medications. 117

How to reduce intermittent fasting side effects 117

HOW LONG DOES IT TAKE FOR INTERMITTENT FASTING TO WORK? 119

Exactly How Much Time Does It Take For Intermittent Fasting To Work 124

Factors that may impact the result Getty 125

Other benefits of intermittent fasting gee 125

CAN I DRINK DURING INTERMITTENT FASTING? 127

Ketosis and Weight Loss 128

Insulin Resistance and Type-2-Diabetes 130

Fasting and Autophagy 131

But how can be determined if a drink stops autophagy? 132

Can You Drink Water During Intermittent Fasting? 134

Can I Drink Carbonated Water During Intermittent Fasting? 136

On the one hand, it offers effects that excellently support intermittent fasting: 136

Can You Drink Flavored Sparkling Water While Intermittent Fasting? 137

Intermittent Fasting and Infused Water 138

Can You Drink Lemon Water During Intermittent Fasting? 139

Can I Drink Coconut Water During Intermittent Fasting? 140

Can You Drink Tea While Intermittent Fasting? 140

Green Tea and Intermittent Fasting 141

Can I Drink Herbal Tea While Intermittent Fasting? ... 143

Ginger and Chai Tea on Intermittent Fasting 144

Can You Drink Milk During Intermittent Fasting? 145

The same applies to cinnamon, which also yields exciting health benefits. 146

   Can You Add Honey to Tea While Fasting? 146

   Tea With Sweetener.. 146

Can You Drink Coffee During Intermittent Fasting?... 147

Black Coffee and Espresso 148

Can You Drink Bulletproof Coffee During Intermittent Fasting? 149

Can I Drink Bone Broth During Intermittent Fasting? 151

Can I Drink Pickle Juice While Intermittent Fasting?... 152

Can You Drink Apple Cider Vinegar During Intermittent Fasting? 153

Can You Drink Juice While Intermittent Fasting?........ 154

   Fasting, Fruit and Vegetable Juice............................. 154

Can You Drink Celery Juice While Intermittent Fasting? 155

Can You Drink Smoothies During Intermittent Fasting? 156

But Can You Drink Lemonade While Fasting? 156

Can You Drink Diet Soda While Intermittent Fasting? 157

Fasting and Diet Coke... 157

   Intermittent Fasting and Coke Zero 158

   Green Coke and Stevia... 159

HOW MUCH WEIGHT CAN YOU LOSE IN A MONTH WITH INTERMITTENT FASTING? 167

Choosing your intermittent fasting plan 168

The 16/8 method 168

The 5:2 method 170

Eat Stop Eat 172

Alternate-day fasting 173

Alternate-day fasting has proven weight loss benefits. 174

The Warrior diet 176

INTERMITTENT FASTING AND THE PHASE 1 DIET FOR MAXIMUM FAT BURNING 178

Fasting For Fat Loss Is Extremely Effective 178

What You Learn About Yourself During Fasting 180

Intermittent Fasting Is A Lifestyle And Not A Diet. 180

What Is The Phase One Diet AKA The Fungus Link? 181

So What Is Allowed On The Phase 1 Diet? 181

PROOF THAT INTERMITTENT FASTING AND BODYBUILDING WORK TOGETHER 184

Proof That Intermittent Fasting and Bodybuilding Work Together 185

Amazing Body 186

Can you emulate him using intermittent fasting? 186

Calorie Surplus for muscle building 187

What works for you? 187

MY EXPERIENCE WITH INTERMITTENT FASTING 188

My Experience With Intermittent Fasting the 5:2 Way 193

Past Eating 193

5:2 Intermittent Fasting 194

Health Benefits and Weight Loss 194

Low Carb But Not Keto 196

What Days To Fast 196

Non-Fast Days 196

Support 197

FREQUENTLY ASKED QUESTIONS, CONCERNS, AND COMPLAINTS 199

I'm a woman. Should I do anything differently? 199

I could never skip breakfast. How do you do it? 200

I thought you were supposed to eat every 3 hours? .. 200

This is crazy. If I didn't eat for 24 hours, I'd die. 202

CONCLUSION 204

Get your free content, **6 healthy recipes for your meal plan.**

Go to the following link: https://bit.ly/3w5SRBr

INTRODUCTION

In the last few years, intermittent fasting has grown in popularity.

Unlike other diets, which rely on when to eat, intermittent fasting emphasizes what to eat by integrating frequent short-term fasts into the daily routine.

This eating style can assist you in consuming fewer calories, losing weight, and lowering your risk of diabetes and heart disease.

Intermittent fasting can seem to be a perfect option for women who want to lose weight, but many people wonder if women should run. Is it possible for women to fast intermittently? A few primary articles on intermittent fasting have been published, and they will help to shed light on this fascinating emerging dietary pattern.

While there are many variants on this diet, intermittent fasting is also known as alternate-day fasting. In a new report published in the American

Journal of Clinical Nutrition, 16 obese men and women participated in a 10-week weight-loss program. Participants ate enough food to meet 25% of their expected energy requirements on fasting days. They were offered nutritional advice for the remainder of the day, but no clear instructions to obey.

The participants did lose weight as planned as a result of the trial, but the researchers were more intrigued by certain specific improvements. After just 10 weeks, the participants were all still obese, but their cholesterol, LDL-cholesterol, triglycerides, and systolic blood pressure levels had improved. The fact that most people ought to lose more weight than the research participants to see the same results made this a fascinating discovery. It was an intriguing discovery that has prompted many people to pursue fasting.

Women will reap certain health benefits from intermittent fasting. It is particularly important for women who are seeking to lose weight because they have a higher fat percentage in their bodies than men. When striving to lose weight, the body burns glucose reserves for the first 6 hours before switching to fat burning. Fasting is a viable option for women who are dealing with stubborn weight despite maintaining a balanced diet and fitness schedule.

Women Over 50 Intermittent Fasting

When we reach menopause, our bodies and metabolisms alter dramatically. One of the most noticeable differences in women over 50 is a sluggish metabolism, which causes them to gain weight. On the other hand, Fasting can be a good way to reverse and avoid this weight gain. According to studies, this fasting pattern tends to suppress appetite, and people who practice it daily don't get the same cravings as others. Intermittent fasting will help you stop eating too much daily if you're over 50 and trying to adapt to your slower metabolism.

When you reach the age of 50, the body begins to experience chronic conditions such as elevated cholesterol and blood pressure. Even without significant weight loss, intermittent fasting has been found to lower cholesterol and blood pressure. If you've seen the figures at the doctor's office increase year after year, you may be able to lower them by fasting, even if you don't lose much weight.

For certain women, intermittent fasting might not be a good option. Anyone should consult a doctor with a specific health condition or who tends to be hypoglycemic. On the other hand, this latest dietary pattern has unique benefits for women who naturally accumulate more fat in their bodies and can struggle to lose it.

How to Quickly Lose Fat for Women

It is possible to lose weight straightforwardly, but it is also possible to lose weight confusingly. Since weight reduction isn't a complicated calculation, it's easy. You will lose weight as long as you consume fewer calories than your body burns. On the other hand, those who don't know how to build the necessary caloric deficiency without depriving or starving themselves can be very frustrating. Regardless of why we want to lose weight, we are ultimately in a race against time. So, these are the easiest ways for women to lose weight easily.

Intermittent Fasting for Fat Loss

For the last few years, the fitness industry has given fasting for weight loss a poor rap. Fasting has many theories and stereotypes about it, and people tend to be afraid of it. Before we proceed, let's dispel those popular misconceptions. Fasting does not put your body into the dreaded "starvation mode," nor does it retard your metabolism or induce muscle breakdown. To keep the metabolism running, the exercise industry makes us believe that we must take regular meals during the day. When we skip a meal or skip breakfast, our bodies go into hunger mode, which slows down our metabolism. This is one of the most common misconceptions in the industry.

It Is Very Difficult to Keep Calories Down

I get the concept of consuming small meals during the day, but the concern is that many people underestimate how many calories each meal contains. When eating in this way, it can be tough to keep the calories down. Instead, eating for 24 hours 1-2 days a week results in a significant calorie deficit without causing harm to the metabolism. This method helps you lose weight and helps you break food addictions and improves the body's capacity to cleanse and purify itself. Remember that some of the world's oldest people fasted at least once a week for the rest of their lives. The most important thing to remember is to eat less. You can't work your way out of a poor diet.

High-Intensity Interval Training Followed with Steady State Cardio

You don't have to spend hours on end on a treadmill or workout bike. When it comes to losing weight, long and tedious cardio has become the rule. High-intensity interval training is required. Not only does it eat a lot more calories than conventional cardio, but it also takes a lot less time. High-intensity interval training, or HIIT, is a form of exercise that involves a brief yet intense effort accompanied by a longer rest time with less effort. HIIT can be incorporated into almost every aerobic unit or exercise. Exercise bikes, cycling, hiking, jumping rope, step climbers, and other similar activities are available. Elliptical computers are the only machines I can rule out. There's an explanation why they're so famous with women. They're incredibly easy! You can't put in enough effort on those computers because they're famously inaccurate at calculating how many calories you've burned.

HIIT Outline

1) Light jog or walk for 1 minute

2) Sprint for 30 seconds

2) *Note: These periods can take 15-20 minutes to complete.*

Steady-State Cardio After HIIT

1) A steady jog or brisk walk for 15-30 minutes.

Note: Workouts that include HIIT and steady-state cardio should be completed 3-5 days a week.

Go Into Each Workout On An Empty Stomach For Max HGH Release

Human growth hormone (HGH) is a term used to describe a hormone produced by the human body. This strong hormone aids in the preservation of muscle mass and the burning of fat. HGH levels will gradually rise as a result of a combination of physical exercise and fasting. HGH can burn fat very quickly if you do not consume any calories 3-4 hours before your workout and wait at least 1-2 hours afterward. Allowing your body to burn extra calories naturally rather than punishing yourself with additional exercise is a much easier way to stay in shape.

A Fat Loss Crash Course

There's nothing wrong with acting rashly for a brief period. If that means avoiding snacks, increasing runs, or missing Sunday brunch, then so be it. You'll be shocked by how quickly your body changes if you can get into the routine of finding new ways to cut calories. Often note the diet accounts for approximately 80% of weight loss. While exercise is highly useful, it can only be used as a supplement to a healthy diet. You'll be light years ahead of conventional weight loss recommendations until you understand the definition. Now that you know how to lose fat easily for women, you will be an inspiration to other women who are trying to lose weight.

INTERMITTENT FASTING FOR FAT LOSS: GOOD OR BAD?

If you may or may not have heard, the title of this article contains some pretty clever wordplay. Today I decided to reflect on the new season, the Holidays. With that in mind, let us take a moment to express our gratitude for all or part of the following. Your car, your money, your ego, your reputation among friends and coworkers, your sneakers, your new hip tech device, and all the other cool stuff we consume all come into play. Alternatively, we might say, "Okay, let's take a chill pill and be grateful for friends, families, loved ones, fitness, roofs above our heads, great opportunities, great and plentiful food, clean water, and an overall awesome community."

When we bear any of the above in mind, it brings the topics we discuss here weekly into context. Now, I'm not trying to minimize the value of this information; rather, I'm trying to put it in its proper context so that we all understand that it's not a life or death situation, but rather something that can be used to improve your overall quality of life in a variety of ways. As a result, we'll be able to assist you in contributing more to the society in which you live.

Intermittent Fasting 101:

Intermittent fasting is a concept that you can or may not be familiar with. It's a quite straightforward dietary intervention that's commonly used and, dare I say, very successfully. It entails categorizing the 24-hour day into two states or categories.

"Fast" -ed or "Fast" -ing state: (Anywhere from 18-48 hours)

"Fed" or "Feed" -ing state

Let's start with your fasting condition. The duration varies between 16 and 48 hours. I've recently experimented with the 16-hour state and had a few encounters with the 24-hour easy.

To begin, your dinner will usually be served around 7:00 or 8:00 p.m. For this case, you will then enter your Fast for the next 16-18 hours. Then you'd get up the next morning, do your morning exercise, and maybe get ready for work.

Side note: If you exercise in the mornings, I will do this once a week rather than on workout days. This is something I like to do on cardio-only days or once a week with Resistance Training exercises.

You should eat the first lunch between 11 a.m. and 1 p.m. on that day.

Things to consider during your fast:

- Potential Irritability
- Increased need for water consumption
- Greater ability to differentiate between false hunger and real hunger
- Great caloric deficit and resetting of the body's fat-burning hormonal environment.
- During a "fasting state," it is essential to consume amino acids (specifically before and after morning "fasted state" workouts.)
- When you come out of a fasted state, you have a greater need for a tasty, well-balanced meal.

Let's take a look at the Feeding situation now.

Based on the last meal for the day, this time period will only last 6-10 hours. It is recommended that you eat your key three meals during this period. Breakfast, aka (Break the Fast), is still served, but it is served later than normal. It does not have to include traditional breakfast foods, but it certainly can if that is your preference.

Each meal will be substantial in size and will last you until the next day.

Things to consider during your Feeding or Fed state:

- If you exercise in the evening, keep carbohydrates mild to minimal for pre-workout meals and then eat a high-carb meal afterward to round out the day and put you in a fed condition.
- Don't gorge yourself on junk food for the first meal after the fast; this will completely undo all of the fast's benefits.
- Ensure that the quantities and sizes of the meals are standard. Always pay attention to your body and wait 15-20 minutes after eating to see if you need additional nourishment. That's how long a meal takes to enter the stomach and its hunger-sensing sensory receptors.

Pros and Cons of Intermittent Fasting + General Guidelines:

- Pro: Create a massive caloric deficit
- Pro: Increases fat & calorie burning
- Pro: Improves the capacity to distinguish between real and false hunger sensations.
- Pro: You are not required to eat every 2-3 hours, which can be inconvenient.
- Pro: Increased metabolism and energy levels
- Cons: Women have a hard time with this diet
- Cons: Takes a little getting used to
- Cons: You may feel flat at times, but this is not something that is commonly stated.

Guidelines:

I don't suggest doing this more than 2-4 times a week, with 2-3 days being my sweet spot right now.

I propose that you give it a shot to see how you react. Every individual is unique.

Get any amino acids on hand and ready to use in the mornings and during and after workouts.

Finally, please seek medical advice before doing something.

That's what there is to it, gentlemen. Give intermittent fasting for weight loss a shot and let me know what you think in the comments section. It really encourages me to simplify things for you when you leave comments and questions.

INTERMITTENT FASTING, ADF, OR 5:2 FASTING IS EFFECTIVE?

If you tried intermittent fasting and had some good results, you should keep doing things your way. However, there is a common and successful approach for getting results that are comparable to or better than conventional fasting. This is known as the 5:2 diet, which means that you regularly consume 5 days a week but only eat a small amount on the other two days. The only difference between an intermittent type and a 5:2 diet is that a 5:2 diet does not require you to limit your food consumption strictly. You essentially regulate your appetite in a systematic and deliberate manner.

Is the 5:2 diet different from intermittent fasting?

Yes, the aim of the 5:2 diet is to help you reduce or offset your extra calorie consumption on weekdays by getting it down to almost zero on the two fasting days. You must be careful not to overeat or eat anything extra on non-fasting days to compensate for the calorie lost on fasting days. It is recommended that you keep your weekday diet to your usual diet since this would negate the intent of dieting or appetite management.

Why choose the 5:2 diet?

One of the most appealing aspects of this diet is that it does not require you to fast on any day. On fasting days, you can consume up to 25% of your daily calories. The average daily calorie intake of a woman is about 2000, which means she will eat up to 500 calories on fast days. Men must limit their calorie intake to 600 on fasting days since the average man consumes approximately 2400 calories per day. Following a full fasting diet is also not as daunting as it seems. You can take three small meals during the day. As a wise dieter, you can eat foods like leafy vegetables and fruits that are filling, natural, and low in calories.

Does 5:2 diet push your body to starvation mode?

Not in the least. In reality, this is one of the reasons why so many people have been successful in losing weight by adopting this diet. Normally, after 36 hours of decreased calorie consumption, the body goes into deprivation mode, although this is not the case on the 5:2 diet. The key is to stop fasting for more than two days in a row. You can choose when you want to hurry and when you want to eat normally. Fasting for two days in a row will put your metabolism into starvation mode, something you should stop if you want to get the best results.

Benefits of 5:2 diet

- An easy and effective fat loss plan
- Improved metabolic health
- Can be continued for long
- Reduces fasting insulin levels in many diabetics
- An effective solution for those who find restricting calories difficult
- No additional or specific food is required
- You can follow it regularly without any side-effects

What to eat and stop and get the most health benefits from intermittent fasting, whether it's 5:2 or some form of fasting, can be tailored to your dietary needs and lifestyle. However, it's essential to keep in mind that you shouldn't go above the maximum calorie intake for snack frequency.

There are different forms of fasting, such as alternating day fasting, 16/8 eating habits, and more, for weight loss and overall health effects, cardio health, and improved digestion, in addition to Intermittent fasting and 5:2 fasting.

INTERMITTENT FASTING VS LOW CARB DIET?

If you want to lose weight, one of the most common diets is the low-carb diet. Low carb diets come in a variety of flavors, from the well-known Atkins diet to The South Beach Diet. Low-carb diets are not new; contrary to popular belief, Dr. Robert Atkins did not invent the idea. Low-carb diets were also pioneered by Herman Tarnower and Herman Taller, two US diet physicians. Jean Anthelme Brillat-Savarin was the first to advocate diets that allowed you to consume beef, certain dairy foods, lettuce, and non-starchy vegetables while limiting or prohibiting foods containing sugar or starch. Doctors and nutritionists are also debating the safest diet for us to pursue to lose weight.

Initial weight loss by pursuing a low-carb diet does decrease body fat, according to the data. Gardner CD, Kiazand A, Alhassan S, et al., in a new review of common diets (Gardner CD, Kiazand A, Alhassan S, et al. The A TO Z Weight Loss Study: a clinical trial compared the Atkins, Zone, Ornish, and LEARN diets for weight loss and associated risk factors in overweight premenopausal people.

JAMA 2007;297:969-77) Over a two-month to six-month stretch, the Atkins diet produced the best weight loss outcomes. This is the kind of material you find in the news on a daily basis. However, the Atkins diet's effects over a 12-month cycle were not as good, and it was no more successful than the other diets in the report.

Based on my familiarity with low-carb dieting, my own opinion is that, while successful in the short term, diets like Atkins are not sustainable in the long run. To reduce body fat and regulate weight, I believe that the way we eat must be sustainable over time, not just for a few weeks. I've tried Atkins, The South Beach Diet, and Fat Flush in the past. I've taken elements from all of these eating programs and incorporate them into my daily routine. I now have a better idea of how processed carbs affect my body, but I also couldn't stick to these plans as a long-term lifestyle shift.

I became a Retired Dieter this year. This ensures that I can no longer hesitate to consume things that I love. I've given up listening to the news on the next trendy diet or fat-loss fad. Every diet has a hook, but at the end of the day, it all boils down to the same thing: we have to eat less in some way. So, what's the answer?

Intermittent fasting has proven to be an important way for me to shed body fat and maintain a healthy weight. Intermittent fasting is essentially incorporating hours of fasting (no food) into your daily routine. You'll have to eat every day, but you'll also have a time of up to 24 hours without food in your schedule. Intermittent fasting, done once or twice a week, helps you lose weight while also allowing you to eat the foods you want. You normally eat on days where you are not fasting. I'm still removing carbohydrates from my diet while following the I.F. lifestyle. I'm cutting carbohydrates for the equivalent of two whole days per week.

We might argue about theory, but I prefer to focus on outcomes. During my first seven weeks of use, I have never seen outcomes like these in 14 years of experimenting with various diet programs. The other important thing is that, unlike my experience with low-carb diets, I have not been limited with Intermittent Fasting, nor have I experienced any cravings for specific items, as I did with low-carb dieting since no foods are forbidden. Why do I believe that after just 7 weeks, I would use intermittent fasting on a long-term basis? The reason is that for every diet I've attempted in the past, I've still felt limited on some days, making the diet impossible to adhere to, and that's on diets that I've managed to stick to for 7 weeks! The distinction in Intermittent Fasting is that it isn't a diet, so it allows you to eat whatever you want. Once you've done one fast, you'll be able to integrate that into your routine going forward; how you do that and how much you do it is entirely up to you; that's the beauty of Intermittent Fasting; it adapts to your lifestyle. How much did you go on a diet in the past, and how much did it affect your life? This is also another example of why diets crash.

Beneficial Low Carb Intermittent Fasting

Low-carbohydrate diets can restrict carbohydrates to 100 or even 50 grams per day. This includes limiting carbohydrates, starches, and other high-carbohydrate items. This is obviously safer for the body because your pancreas may not have to work as hard to extract sugars from your system.

Fasting over a set period of time is known as intermittent fasting (many people fast 24 hours then eat healthy the next 24 hours, and so on). This means your body needs to scavenge for food (fuel) and, in the end, eliminates old or dead cells as well as any waste that has accumulated in your body.

As you combine the two for "Low Carb Intermittent Fasting," you'll have a winning formula for losing weight and looking fantastic.

You should drink low-carb, low-calorie beverages like water and black coffee when fasting, so you can not eat for more than 24 hours. The next day, you can typically eat, but you should also limit your carbohydrate intake. To ensure you're making the right decisions for your body and fitness, read labels and review foods.

New or "live" foods are often excellent options. Remember that what goes in must come out and that making better decisions leads to a happier lifestyle. This is a lifestyle improvement that can be maintained for the rest of your life (at least the low carbs). You must make a conscious decision to consume healthy foods and beverages!

When you combine low-carb intermittent fasting with exercise, you'll be in shape and feeling great in no time.

Fasting for short periods prevents fat oxidation and can help you lose weight. Exercising can hasten the process and aid in the removal of flabby skin and toning.

Intermittent fasting has been shown to extend the lifetime of animals by 40 percent or more. That's incredible! This demonstrates how eating well and cleaning your body will support your system and aid in weight loss and your days on this planet.

Vegetables are a low-carb food choice. You are free to consume as many vegetables as you desire. Dinner options include meats and seafood. Create a salad with a fried egg, tomato, and a pinch of cheese for lunch. However, keep an eye on the calories in the dressing.

Your appetite for sugars and carbs will most likely vanish as long as you are committed to making healthier lifestyle choices. The appetite will undoubtedly dwindle! When you make the decision to consume nutritious, low-carb meals, you can no longer crave greasy, sweet foods.

Also, drink plenty of water. Black coffee and green tea are both decent options, please don't go overboard on the caffeine. Always consult with your health care provider before beginning any diet or workout regimen! You want to make sure you remain safe while you improve your fitness!

INTERMITTENT FASTING SCHEDULE

If you're thinking of giving fasting a try, you have a few choices for incorporating it into your daily routine.

Daily Intermittent Fasting

I usually adopt the Leangains intermittent fasting style, which involves a 16–hour fast accompanied by an 8–hour feeding cycle. Martin Berkhan of Leangains.com popularized this style of frequent intermittent fasting, which is where the name came from.

It makes no difference when you begin your eight-hour feeding time. You will begin at 8 a.m. and end at 4 p.m. Alternatively, you could begin at 2 p.m. and end at 10 p.m.

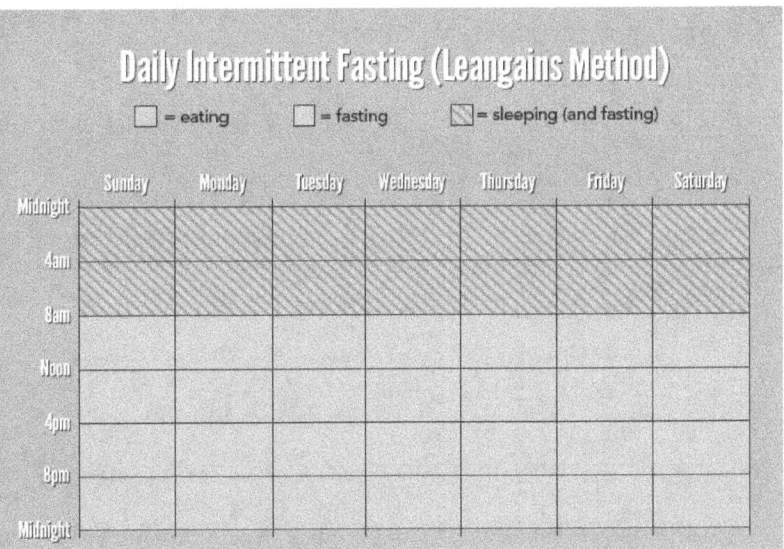

What works for you is what you can do. I notice that eating between 1 and 8 p.m. fits well for me because it allows me to have lunch and dinner with friends and family. Breakfast is usually a meal I eat alone, so skipping it isn't a huge deal for me.

It's very straightforward to fall into the routine of eating on this schedule when regular intermittent fasting is done every day. You're actually eating at the same time every day right now without even realizing it. It's the same thing with regular intermittent fasting; you simply learn not to feed at some hours, which is surprisingly easy.

A theoretical drawback of this schedule is that when you usually skip a meal or two during the day, getting the same amount of calories during the week becomes more complicated. Simply put, it's difficult to train yourself to consume larger meals on a regular basis. As a result, many people who experiment with this form of extended fasting lose weight. Depending on your objectives, this can be a positive or negative thing.

This is also an excellent time to point out that, while I've been doing intermittent fasting for the past year, I'm not a diet zealot. I focus on developing healthier behaviors that control my actions 90% of the time so that I can do anything I want with the remaining 10%. Guess what happens if I come over to your house to watch the football game and we order pizza at 11 p.m.? I don't care if it's outside of my feeding window; I'm going to eat it.

Weekly Intermittent Fasting

Once a week or once a month is one of the easiest ways to get acquainted with intermittent fasting. Even if you don't use fasting to cut calories on a regular basis, the occasional fast has been found to contribute to all of the effects of fasting we've already discussed, so there are still many other health benefits of fasting.

The diagram below depicts one possible scenario for a weekly sporadic fast.

Lunch on Monday, for example, is your last meal of the day. Then you fast until Tuesday lunchtime. This routine gives you the option of eating any day of the week while also getting the advantages of fasting for 24 hours. Since you're just taking out two meals a week, it's much less likely that you'll lose weight. So, whether you want to bulk up or maintain your weight, this is a perfect choice.

I've done 24-hour fasts before (most recently last month), and there are many combinations and choices for fitting it into your timetable. A long day of driving, for example, or the day after a large holiday feast are also excellent opportunities to incorporate a 24-hour fast.

Perhaps the most significant advantage of a 24-hour fast is overcoming the emotional hurdle of fasting. If you've never fasted before, finishing the first one will make you remember that going without food for a day won't kill you.

Alternate Day Intermittent Fasting

Alternate day extended fasting involves fasting for longer stretches of time on several days throughout the week.

In the diagram below, you will eat dinner on Monday night and then not eat again until Tuesday evening. On Wednesday, though, you will eat all day and then resume the 24-hour fasting time after dinner. This encourages you to maintain long fast stretches while consuming at least one meal every day of the week.

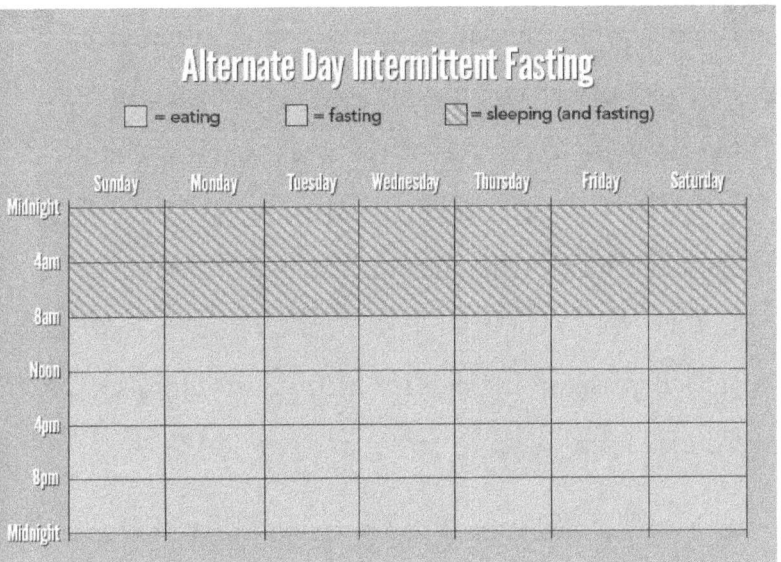

According to what I've seen, this kind of intermittent fasting seems to be common in scientific studies, but it isn't very popular in the real world. I've never attempted alternate-day fasting and have no plans to do so in the future.

Alternate-day intermittent fasting has the advantage of allowing you to stay in a fasted state for longer than the Leangains method. This, in theory, would boost the effects of fasting.

In reality, however, I'd be nervous about not eating enough. In my view, one of the most daunting facets of intermittent fasting is training oneself to eat more often. You may be able to feast for a meal, but doing so every day of the week requires a little planning, a lot of cooking, and consistent feeding. As a result, most people who attempt intermittent fasting lose weight while the size of their meals stays consistent despite the fact that a few meals are skipped each week.

This isn't a challenge if you're trying to lose weight.

And if you're satisfied with your weight, if you stick to the regular or weekly fasting routines, this won't be too much of a problem. However, if you're fasting for 24 hours a day on several days a week, it'll be impossible to compensate for adequate food on your feast days.

As a result, I believe that trying occasional intermittent fasting or a single 24-hour fast once a week or once a month is a smarter option.

Intermittent fasting can be done in a variety of ways. The number of fast days and calorie allowances differ between the systems.

Intermittent fasting entails going without food for a period of time, either completely or partly, before eating normally again.

According to some research, this type of eating will help you lose weight, improve your fitness, and live longer. Intermittent fasting advocates argue that it is simpler to stick to than conventional calorie-controlled diets.

Intermittent fasting is a personal experience for each person, and different styles will serve other people.

Seven ways to do intermittent fasting

Intermittent fasting can be done in a variety of ways, though different people choose different forms. Continue reading to learn about seven different ways to quick intermittently.

1. Fast for 12 hours a day

The diet's guidelines are straightforward. Every day, a person must choose and follow a 12-hour fasting window.

According to some researchers, fasting for 10–16 hours causes the body to convert fat reserves into energy, releasing ketones into the bloodstream. This should help you lose weight.

For beginners, this form of intermittent fasting strategy may be a reasonable choice. This is due to the fact that the fasting window is comparatively short, much of the fasting happens while sleeping, and the individual will eat the same amount of calories per day.

The most convenient way to complete the 12-hour fast is to include sleep time in the fasting window.

An individual might, for example, fast between the hours of 7 p.m. and 7 a.m. They'd have to end dinner until 7 p.m. and wait before 7 a.m. to eat breakfast, but they'd be sleeping for the majority of the time in between.

2. Fasting for 16 hours

The 16:8 cycle, also known as the Leangains diet, involves fasting for 16 hours a day and only feeding for 8 hours.

Men fast for 16 hours a day and women fast for 14 hours on the 16:8 diet. This method of intermittent fasting could be beneficial for those who have attempted the 12-hour fast and found it to be ineffective.

People who fast this way typically finish their evening meal by 8 p.m., miss breakfast the next day, and don't eat again until noon.

Even though mice consumed the same total amount of calories as mice that ate anytime they wanted, reducing the feeding window to 8 hours saved them from obesity, inflammation, diabetes, and liver disease, according to a source.

3. Fasting for 2 days a week

The 5:2 diet requires people to consume a normal amount of healthy food for five days and then decrease their calorie consumption for the next two days.

Men usually eat 600 calories and women 500 calories over the two fasting days.

Fasting days are usually separated during the week. They can, for example, fast on Mondays and Thursdays and normally eat for the rest of the week. On fasting days, there should be at least one non-fasting day.

The 5:2 diet, also known as the Fast diet, has received little research. A study of 107 overweight or obese people discovered that calorie restriction twice weekly and constant calorie restriction also resulted in similar weight loss.

The diet also reduced insulin levels and improved insulin sensitivity in the participants, according to the study.

The results of this fasting type on 23 overweight women were studied in a small-scale analysis. The women lost 4.8 percent of their body weight and

8.0 percent of their excess body fat in one menstrual cycle. After 5 days of the regular diet, the majority of the women's measurements returned to normal.

4. Alternate day fasting

The alternate-day fasting plan, which includes fasting every other day, has many variants.

Some people practice alternate-day fasting by avoiding solid foods entirely on fasting days, while others accommodate up to 500 calories. People always want to eat as much as they want on feeding days.

According to One Source, alternate fasting is successful for weight loss and heart well-being in both lean and overweight people. Over the course of a 12-week cycle, the 32 participants lost an average of 5.2 kilograms (kg), or just over 11 pounds (lb).

Alternate-day fasting is a more severe type of intermittent fasting that may not be appropriate for beginners or people with certain medical conditions. This method of fasting can also be difficult to sustain over time.

5. A weekly 24-hour fast

The Eat-Stop-Eat diet entails going without food for 24 hours at a time for one to two days a week. Many people fast from one meal to the next or from one meal to the next.

People on this diet plan will drink wine, tea, and other calorie-free beverages during the fasting time.

On non-fasting days, people should resume their daily eating habits. This way of eating lowers a person's overall calorie consumption, leaving the individual's food choices unrestricted.

Fasting for 24 hours can be difficult, as it can lead to nausea, headaches, and irritability. As the body responds to this new eating routine, many people feel that these symptoms become less severe with time.

Before attempting the 24-hour fast, people can profit from attempting a 12-hour or 16-hour fast.

6. Meal skipping

Beginners can benefit from this versatile approach to intermittent fasting. It entails missing meals on occasion.

People will choose which meals to miss based on their hunger levels or time constraints. It is, however, important to consume nutritious foods at - meal.

Individuals who track and respond to their bodies' hunger signals are more likely to succeed at meal skipping. People who practice intermittent fasting in this manner eat when they are hungry and miss meals when they are not.

For certain people, this may sound more normal than the other fasting approaches.

7. The Warrior Diet

The Warrior Diet is a form of intermittent fasting that is very severe.

During a 20-hour fasting time, the Warrior Diet entails consuming very little, typically only a few portions of raw fruit and vegetables, and only enjoying one full meal at night. In most cases, the feeding time is just 4 hours long.

This form of intermittent fasting could be better for people who have already experienced other types of intermittent fasting.

The Warrior Diet advocates argue that humans are normal nocturnal eaters and that feeding at night helps the body to gain nutrients according to its circadian rhythms.

People can make sure to eat lots of greens, meats, and healthy fats over the 4-hour feeding period. Carbohydrates can also be used.

Although it is possible to consume certain foods during the fasting time, adhering to the rigid rules for when and when to eat in the long run can be difficult. Furthermore, some people find it difficult to consume such a big meal so close to bedtime.

There's even a chance that people on this diet won't get enough nutrients like fiber. This will raise cancer risk and have a negative impact on digestive and immune function.

Tips for maintaining intermittent fasting
Maintaining an intermittent fasting regimen can be difficult.

The following suggestions will help people keep on track and get the most out of intermittent fasting:

- **Staying hydrated.** Throughout the day, drink plenty of water and calorie-free beverages like herbal teas.
- **Avoiding obsessing over food.** On fasting days, plan many distractions to keep you from worrying about food, such as catching up on paperwork or seeing a movie.
- **Resting and relaxing.** On fasting days, avoid strenuous exercises, while light exercises such as yoga can be helpful.
- **Making every calorie count.** Choose nutrient-dense meals that are high in protein, fiber, and healthy fats if the preferred schedule requires any calories during fasting times. Corn, lentils, eggs, chicken, almonds, and avocado are only a few examples.
- **Eating high-volume foods.** Choose foods that are both filling and low in calories, such as popcorn, raw vegetables, and fruits with

high water content, such as grapes and melon.

Increasing flavor without adding calories. Garlic, vegetables, sauces, or vinegar may be used liberally to season meals. These foods are very low in calories but high in taste, which can help to alleviate hunger pangs.

After the fasting time, use nutrient-dense foods. Consuming diets rich in fiber, vitamins, minerals, and other nutrients helps maintain blood sugar levels and avoid nutritional deficiencies. A well-balanced diet can help you lose weight and improve your general health.

INTERMITTENT FASTING MEAL PLANS

Whenever a new food pattern enters the public consciousness, I want to give it a shot. I've done it all: Whole30, South Beach, Paleo, Vegan, you name it. I've been reading a lot about Intermittent Fasting (IF) lately. Although it isn't a brand-new way of living, it is getting a moment and gaining traction in the health community.

At first, I felt apprehensive. Breakfast, I've been told for years, is the most critical meal of the day. Now I'm hearing that you should miss breakfast each day and wait as long as possible before feeding. Isn't it sending mixed messages?

After doing some research into the specifics, as well as the benefits and drawbacks of IF, I decided to give it a try. As I navigated IF for the first time, Sarah discussed some of the benefits of IF, including increased vitality, weight loss (if weight loss is desired), and enhanced blood lipids and glucose balance.

For the past month, I've been experimenting with IF and am able to share my reflections and insights with you.

Let's begin with the various forms of fasting. According to my study, four forms of IF stand out as the most popular:

- Fast for 14 to 16 hours (women) and then eat for the last eight to ten hours.
- Normally eat five days a week and just about 1/4 of the daily calorie intake on the other two days (known as the 5:2 plan).
- Quick for a full 24 hours once or twice a week.
- Fast for the majority of the day and only eat one meal at night.

For me, just the first and second choices seemed to be even vaguely feasible. I experimented with all forms over the course of my four-week trial.

For weeks one and two, I followed the 5:2

schedule, and for weeks three and four, I followed the 14 hours easy / 10-hour feeding plan.

Weeks One and Two: The 5:2 Plan

This strategy was pretty simple for me to execute. It was important to schedule out my two days of limited eating at the start of each week. This was crucial in order for me to avoid having to skip out on arrangements with colleagues. Planning has helped me physically prepare for those challenging low-calorie days.

In terms of workouts, I decided to do lighter workouts in the mornings of my low-calorie days before I became hungry. I prepared my kitchen by filling my fridge with low-calorie foods, focusing on vegetables since a serving of 10 cups contains 500 calories. I snacked on cucumbers and tomatoes, drank plenty of water, and drank coffee and tea throughout the day. To keep my energy levels high when I got hungry, I definitely drank too much coffee during these days. I assume that if I kept to this diet for a longer period of time, I would get used to the feels of low-calorie days and would be less reliant on coffee or green tea.

During the low-calorie days, I was starving, but nothing I couldn't handle. It wasn't so bad as long as I could snack on vegetables and drink plenty of water. The next day, I still noticed the consequences of the low-calorie day. I awoke feeling light, and if there is such a thing as the opposite of bloated, that's how I felt. It was fantastic! But the next day, I was exhausted. My exercises didn't struggle the day of the low-calorie eating (I usually exercise before eating anyway), but they did the next day. If I kept this strategy, I would do my lighter workouts the day after my low-calorie day.

Weeks Three and Four: 14 Hours Fasting / 10 Hours Eating Plan

I changed my schedule for these weeks. I fasted for 14 hours a day (eight of which are when you're sleeping!) and then fed for 10 hours a day. My greatest challenge was maintaining healthier eating habits over my 10-hour meal period. It's quick to fall into the trap of thinking that while you've been limiting yourself, you can eat whatever you want when the time comes. It is not the point of the software, and it is impossible that you can achieve success if you do so.

The tension of planning for the fast or getting off the fast was another issue with this strategy. I was either worried about fasting and how hungry I'd be, or I overate before the fast. Then it was time to eat as soon as my fast was over. Since I felt like I deserved it, I let my guard down more than usual. Sleeping late made this possible, but sleeping as late as possible to reduce the awake fasting time doesn't make for a very efficient day.

This schedule was more difficult for me to stick to because it affected every single day, while the 5:2 plan only affected two days a week. When proposals arose, it was more difficult to adhere to this schedule.

Beyond the Fasting Window

As critical as the fasting window is, Sarah emphasizes the importance of eating the right foods to break the fast. She suggests a diet that is rich in protein and fat but low in carbohydrates. This allows you to feel satisfied without causing a blood sugar spike. Nuts, cheese, whole fat pure greek yogurt, or steel-cut oatmeal with nuts and seeds are among Sarah's favorite ways to split the quick. Sarah suggests eating a big breakfast after a fast, around a quarter of your daily calories.

Next Steps: Will I Stick With IF?

Moving forward, I don't want to live an IF lifestyle 100 percent of the time, but there were certainly takeaways from my IF experience.

Hunger cues were one of the most important things I learned from this experience. These four weeks helped me to reconnect with my hunger signals, which I had been ignoring for far too long. Many of us eat for a number of reasons, not just because we are starving. Sarah and I discussed how it's normal for people to disregard hunger signals and eat when they're bored when someone else is feeding, when food is in front of them when they're stressed, and so on. My IF experience taught me what it's like to be hungry and how important it is to pay attention to those clues. I'm notorious for eating out of hunger, and I'm hoping that a greater sense of when I'm genuinely hungry will help me reduce this.

Here are the biggest takeaways from my IF experience:

It doesn't have to be either/or. If I didn't meet my 14-hour fasting target, I felt like I had failed. Sarah reminded me that every improvement is a step in the right direction; you don't have to be flawless all of the time. But it's fine if you can do the 14-hour easy one day but not the next because of your timetable. Don't give up on IF because you can't keep it up 100% of the time.

Experiment with different options to see what fits best for you. Since different styles fit best on other individuals, there are other forms of IF. Try them all, or whatever sounds perfect before choosing one you can stay with and be happy with.

Finding a groove takes time. This is true with every new routine or habit, not just IF. Cut yourself some slack if it's difficult at first; you're always getting your bearings. Be mindful that adjusting to a new schedule and routine can take time.

Get up! This is true to IF as well as the majority of other good behaviors. The more trained you are, the more likely you are to succeed.

Hydration is Key: This should go without saying,

but it never hurts to be reminded. If you're fasting (which is especially important!) or not, make sure you're getting enough water.

Do you want to try Intermittent Fasting? Most people can safely try IF. It is not recommended, though, if you have a history of disordered eating. Consult your doctor before beginning any drug that alters your metabolism (especially diabetes medications) or allows you to consume food. If you're not sure if IF is right for you, talk to your doctor or a registered dietitian before starting a program.

What Foods Are Best to Eat on an Intermittent Fasting Diet?

- Before making any major dietary changes, consult with a wellness provider to ensure that it is the right choice for you.
- Intermittent fasting (IF) is making quite an uproar in the overcrowded world of dieting, including the word "fasting" sounding ominous.
- A fair amount of evidence (albeit with small sample sizes) shows that the diet can help people lose weight and control their blood sugar levels. It's no surprise that everyone and their aunt have jumped on the IF bandwagon.
- The absence of diet guidelines can be appealing: there are limitations on what you can eat, but not actually when you may eat.
- Though, it's still necessary to consider what's at stake. Should you be breaking your fast with pints of ice cream and bags of chips? Very likely not. That's why we've compiled a list of the best things to eat on an IF diet.

So WTF should I eat on IF?

Lauren Harris-Pincus, MS, RDN, author of The Protein-Packed Breakfast Club, says, "There are no specifications or limitations on what kind or how much food to consume when practicing intermittent fasting."

Lauren Harris-Pincus, MS, RDN, author of The Protein-Packed Breakfast Club, says, "There are no specifications or limitations on what kind or how much food to consume when practicing intermittent fasting."

However, Mary Purdy, MS, RDN, chair of Dietitians of Integrative and Functional Medicine, counters that "the effects [of IF] are unlikely to follow consistent Big Mac meals."

According to Pincus and Purdy, a well-balanced diet is a secret to gaining weight, retaining energy levels, and keeping to the diet.

"Anyone trying to lose weight should eat nutrient-dense foods like fruits, vegetables, whole grains, nuts, beans, seeds, dairy, and lean proteins," Pincus recommends.

"My guidelines will be somewhat similar to the foods I would usually prescribe for better health —

high-fiber, unprocessed, whole foods that provide variety and flavor," Purdy says.

To put it another way, if you consume a lot of the foods mentioned below, you won't get hungry while fasting.

1. Water

Okay, so this isn't actually a snack, but it's incredibly necessary for surviving IF.

Water is important for the protection of almost all of your body's main organs. Avoiding this as part of the fast would be stupid. Your lungs play a critical role in keeping you alive.

The amount of water that each person can drink depends on their gender, height, weight, level of exercise, and environment. However, the color of the urine is a good indicator. For all times, you like it to be pale yellow.

Dehydration, which may induce headaches, nausea, and lightheadedness, is indicated by dark yellow urine. When you combine it with a lack of calories, you have a recipe for catastrophe — or, at the very least, really dark pee.

If plain water doesn't appeal to you, try adding a splash of lemon juice, a few mint leaves, or cucumber slices to it.

Here's why H2O is the champion.

2. Avocado

Eating the highest-calorie fruit when attempting to lose weight can appear counterintuitive. On the other hand, avocados will hold you full through even the most stringent fasting times thanks to their high unsaturated fat content.

Unsaturated fats, according to research, help keep the body healthy even though you don't feel hungry. Your body sends out signals that it doesn't need to go into emergency hunger mode because it has enough calories. And if you're starving in the midst of a fasting time, unsaturated fats keep these symptoms running much longer.

Another research showed that using half an

avocado in your lunch will help you stay full for hours longer than if you don't eat the green, mushy fruit.

3. Fish and seafood

There's an explanation why the American Dietary Guidelines recommend two or three 4-ounce servings of fish every week.

In addition to being high in good fats and proteins, it is also high in vitamin D.

And if you like to feed at short window times, don't you want to get more nutritious bang for your buck when you do?

You'll never run out of ways to prepare fish because there are so many options.

4. Cruciferous veggies

The f-word — fiber — is abundant in foods like broccoli, brussels sprouts, and cauliflower. (We see what you're saying, and no, the f-word doesn't stand for "farts.")

It's important to eat fiber-rich foods at frequent intervals to keep you regular and ensure that your poop factory runs smoothly.

Fiber will also help you feel whole, which is beneficial if you won't be able to eat for another 16 hours.

Cruciferous vegetables can also help you avoid cancer.

5. Potatoes

Repeat after us: White foods aren't all evil.

In the 1990s, the researchers discovered that potatoes were one of the most satiating foods. In addition, a 2012 study showed that using potatoes in a balanced diet can aid weight loss. (Sorry, but potato chips and french fries don't count.)

We looked into the relationship between potatoes and blood sugar.

5. Beans and legumes

On the IF diet, your favorite chili topping could be

your best friend.

Food, specifically carbohydrates, provides energy for physical activity. We're not suggesting you go crazy with carbohydrates, but including low-calorie carbs like beans and legumes in your diet can't hurt. This will help you stay awake through your fasting period.

Furthermore, foods like chickpeas, black beans, peas, and lentils have been shown to help people lose weight even when they aren't on a diet.

6. Probiotics

What do the little critters in your stomach want to eat the most? Both consistency and variety are essential. When they're starving, this means they're not comfortable. And if your stomach isn't comfortable, you might notice any unpleasant side effects, such as constipation.

Add probiotic-rich ingredients to your diets, such as kefir, kombucha, and sauerkraut, to combat this unpleasantness.

We spoke to specialists to learn more about how probiotics function in the body.

7. Berries

These smoothie classics are packed with vitamins and minerals. That's not even the most exciting aspect.

People who ate a lot of flavonoids, such as those used in blueberries and strawberries, had lower BMI rises over 14 years than people who didn't eat berries, according to a 2016 report.

8. Eggs

One big egg has 6.24 grams of protein and takes just minutes to prepare. And, particularly when you're eating less, having as much protein as possible is critical for staying full and building muscle.

Men who had an egg breakfast instead of a bagel were less hungry and ate less during the day, according to a 2010 survey.

To put it another way, if you're looking for something to do during your quick, why not hard-boil a bunch of eggs? And, when the time is right, you should eat them.

9. Nuts

While nuts are higher in calories than many other snacks, they do have something that most snacks do not: healthy fats.

Even don't be concerned with calories! According to a 2012 report, a 1-ounce serving of almonds (roughly 23 nuts) contains 20% fewer calories than the label claims.

Chewing does not fully break down the cell walls of almonds, according to the report. Which keeps a part of the nut intact and prevents it from being absorbed by the body during digestion. As a result, eating almonds might not make as much of a difference in your daily calorie intake as you would think.

10. Whole grains

Dieting and carbohydrate use tend to fall into two distinct categories. This isn't always the case, as you'll be glad to learn. Since whole grains are high in fiber and protein, a small amount would keep you satisfied for a long time.

So get out of your comfort zone and try farro, bulgur, spelled, Kamut, amaranth, millet, sorghum, or freekeh, a whole-grain utopia.

WHAT MAKES INTERMITTENT FASTING WORK?

Intermittent fasting (IF) is a dietary eating practice that involves not eating for a long period of time or seriously limiting calories. There are several different types of intermittent fasting, each with its own length of fast; others are for hours, while some are for days (s). Owing to all of the possible exercise and health advantages that are being found, this has become a very common subject in the scientific world.

WHAT IS INTERMITTENT FASTING (IF)?

Fasting, or times of voluntary dietary abstinence, has been observed for centuries all around the world. Intermittent fasting for the sake of bettering one's well being is a relatively recent concept. Intermittent fasting entails limiting your food consumption for a fixed amount of time without making any adjustments to the foods you consume. The most popular IF protocols are a regular 16-hour fast and a one- or two-day fast once or twice a week. Intermittent fasting is a normal feeding practice that humans were designed to follow and can be traced all the way back to our paleolithic hunter-gatherer forefathers. The latest model of a proposed intermittent fasting regimen has the ability to enhance many facets of fitness, including body structure, lifespan, and aging. About the fact that IF goes against our culture's and everyday routines, science might be pointing to less meal frequency and more time fasting as the best solution to the traditional breakfast, lunch, and dinner model. The following are two widespread misconceptions about intermittent fasting.

Myth 1 - This "law" that is universal in Western culture was not established based on evidence for good health but was accepted as the standard pattern for settlers and gradually became the norm. Not only does the three-meal-a-day approaches lack empirical support, but new research suggests that fewer meals and more fasting could be better for human wellbeing. One research found that eating one meal a day of the same number of calories as three meals a day is healthier for weight loss and body health than eating three meals a day. This discovery is a simple principle that can be extrapolated into intermittent fasting. Those who want to do IF can find that eating only 1-2 meals per day is the better option.

Myth 2 - Breakfast is essential since it is the most important meal of the day: Many false assumptions have been made on the sheer necessity of eating breakfast every day. "Breakfast raises the metabolism" and "breakfast reduces food consumption later in the day" are two of the most popular arguments. These arguments have been debunked and studied over a 16-week stretch, with findings indicating that missing breakfast did not lower metabolism or improve food consumption at lunch and dinner. It is still possible to follow intermittent fasting protocols while eating breakfast. Still, some people prefer to eat a late breakfast or skip it entirely, and this common misconception should be dispelled.

TYPES OF INTERMITTENT FASTING:

Intermittent fasting appears in a variety of ways, each with its own range of advantages. The fasting-to-eating ratio varies depending on the type of intermittent fasting. The advantages and efficacy of these various protocols can vary depending on the user, so it's crucial to figure out which one is better for you. Health priorities, regular schedule/routine, and current health status are all factors that can affect which one to select. Alternate-day fasting, time-restricted feeding, and adapted fasting are the most common forms of IF.

1. ALTERNATE DAY FASTING:

This method entails combining days of almost no calories (from food or beverage) with days of unlimited feeding and eating.

Weight reduction, improved blood cholesterol and triglyceride (fat) levels, and improved signals for inflammation in the blood have also been seen to benefit from this strategy.

The biggest disadvantage of this form of intermittent fasting is that it is the most difficult to maintain due to confirmed hunger on fasting days.

2. MODIFIED FASTING - 5:2 DIET

Modified fasting is a regimen that has pre-programmed fasting days but allows for any food consumption on certain days. On fasting days, you are allowed to consume 20-25 percent of your daily calories; for example, if you usually consume 2000 calories on ordinary eating days, you are allowed to consume 400-500 calories on fasting days. The 5:2 ratio corresponds to the number of non-fasting days to fasting days in this diet. So, under this plan, you'd eat regularly for 5 days, then fast or limit calories to 20-25 percent for 2 days.

This protocol is beneficial for weight loss, body structure, and blood sugar, lipids, and inflammation control. The 5:2 protocol has been shown in studies to be beneficial for weight loss, improving/lowering inflammatory markers in the blood (3), and showing signs of insulin resistance improvement. This updated fasting 5:2 diet resulted in lower fat levels, lower appetite hormones (leptin), and higher levels of protein linked to fat burning and blood sugar control in animal tests (adiponectin).

The changed 5:2 fasting regimen is simple to adopt and has only a few undesirable side effects, such as hunger, reduced energy, and irritability when first starting out. Despite this, studies have found benefits such as decreased anxiety, less frustration, less exhaustion, increased self-confidence, and a more optimistic mood.

3. TIME-RESTRICTED FEEDING:

If you meet someone who claims to practice intermittent fasting, it's almost always in the form of time-restricted eating. This is a regular form of intermittent fasting that includes only eating calories for a limited portion of the day and fasting for the rest. In time-restricted eating, daily fasting periods will vary from 12 to 20 hours, with 16/8 being the most common process (fasting for 16 hours, consuming calories for 8). The time of day doesn't matter for this regimen as long as you're fasting for a long period of time and only eating when you're allowed to. On a 16/8 time-restricted feeding program, for example, one person might eat their first meal at 7 a.m. and last meal at 3 p.m. (fast from 3 p.m. to 7 a.m.), while another might eat their first meal at 1 p.m. and last meal at 9 p.m. (fast from 9 PM-1 PM). This protocol is designed to be followed every day for a long time and is very adaptable as long as you remain inside the fasting/eating window (s).

One of the most simple strategies of intermittent fasting is time-restricted eating. This, combined with your regular work and sleep schedule, can assist you in achieving optimal metabolic function.

Time-restricted eating is a perfect regimen to pursue if you want to lose weight and change your body shape and gain some other health benefits. Important weight loss, fasting blood glucose drops, and cholesterol improvements were seen in the few human studies performed, with no increases in perceived tension, exhaustion, frustration, fatigue, or uncertainty. Other preliminary animal research found that time-restricted feeding protects against obesity, elevated insulin, fatty liver disease, and inflammation.

Time-restricted feeding can be an excellent choice for weight loss and chronic disease prevention/management due to its ease of use and positive outcomes. When starting out with this regimen, start with a lower fasting-to-eating ratio, such as 12/12 hours, and gradually work your way up to 16/8 hours.

COMMON QUESTION ABOUT INTERMITTENT FASTING:

Is there any food or drink that I can have during intermittent fasting? You shouldn't eat or drink anything with calories unless you're following the adjusted fasting 5:2 diet (mentioned above). You should drink water, black coffee, and some other non-calorie foods or drinks during fasting time. In reality, sufficient water consumption is needed during IF, and some people believe that drinking black coffee while fasting helps to reduce hunger.

IF YOU JUST WANT THE BENEFITS:
Intermittent fasting research is only in its early stages, but it has enormous potential for weight loss and the prevention of some chronic diseases.

To recap, here are the possible benefits of intermittent fasting:
Shown in Human Studies:

1. Weight loss

2. Improve blood lipid markers like cholesterol

3. Reduce inflammation

4. Reduced stress and improved self-confidence

5. Improved mood

Shown in Animal Studies:

1. Decreased Body Fat

2. Decreased levels of the hunger hormone leptin

3. Improve insulin levels

4. Protect against obesity, fatty liver disease, and inflammation

5. Longevity

There are moments when losing weight seems to necessitate wading through pages of detail, the majority of which contradict one another. One encourages you to eat more, and the other encourages you to eat less. One says you can do cardio for at least an hour a day, and the other says it won't help you lose weight. The grapefruit diet, the banana diet, the golden law of eating breakfast every morning, and the terror of going into hunger mode are only a few examples.

And it's just becoming more difficult by the day.

That's where intermittent fasting's versatility comes in. It's adaptable. It's straightforward. There are certain guidelines to observe, such as not counting calories or obsessing over meals. Most dieters struggle because they see it as a one-time experience, whereas intermittent fasting is a way of life.

It's also a very attainable one, thanks to its versatility and stability.

It acts like this: you swift for a few days a week. It could include 1-3 24-hour fasts every week. Others will have to fast for 15 to 19 hours per day.

To say that it is easy is an understatement. If you've been practicing the often promoted six-meal-a-day diet, you're certainly aware of how much effort is spent planning your meals each day — endlessly obsessing about the time and the next meal, even rearranging your life to suit the diet.

Losing weight with the versatile method of intermittent fasting ensures that your life does not revolve around meals. Rather than scheduling meals around your day, you're scheduling meals around your schedule. You can eat 3,000 calories on non-fasting days if you like, but it only leaves you with a daily calorie intake of 1,500.

Even better, during your fasting days, you can consume as much nutritious food as you want. Veggies, seeds, nutritious proteins and fats, and more are included. However, in the case of refined, high-calorie foods, a judgment call is always required. It's a non-restrictive diet, but it's not a cure-all, and, as in everything else, balance is the secret to success.

Intermittent fasting has been shown to help your well-being in various ways, including keeping your metabolism high, maintaining bone density, increasing fatty acid oxidation, and increasing human growth hormones, among other things.

Fasting as a weight-loss method has recently sparked a lot of controversy and conversation on the internet. Fasting, in my opinion, will help people lose weight and improve their fitness. Intermittent fasting appears to have the ability to lower blood pressure, improve insulin sensitivity, restrict oxidative stress, aid muscle tissue recovery, and aid fat loss, according to research.

Fasting's tendency to do both of these activities may be due to the fact that when the body reaches a fasting mode and there are fewer calories in the environment, the body initiates a sequence of restorative processes that will not be activated in the presence of vast amounts of food. Instead of participating in cell division or creation, the body is more able to restore and revive weakened tissues, requiring less energy and calories. In the process, the body adjusts, tissues and cells repair themselves and become more resilient. According to research done on rodents, a lower-calorie diet contributes to a longer life.

THE FACT THAT FASTING FOR WEIGHT LOSS IS SO SUCCESSFUL HAS TWO MAIN REASONS.

1. Fat burning will occur if there is little to no food in the body.

The body is required to use stored energy sources whether there is little or no fat, protein, or sugar in the bloodstream. Fats contained in tissues and carbohydrates stored in the muscles and liver are examples of those outlets. If you don't fast for an extended period of time, you will lose a lot of weight without putting in a lot of work by skipping a meal or going without eating for a day or two.

2. Fasting Is A Simple Way To Reduce Calories Without Forgoing The Foods You Enjoy.

Though it may be perplexing, skipping one or two meals drastically reduces daily caloric consumption. As a result, as long as you don't overeat, it's perfectly acceptable to eat some of your favorite foods while still eating fewer calories overall for the time period in question.

However, keep in mind the value of ensuring that your fasting is consistent with your lifestyle. I started intermittent fasting a few months ago and have found that it helps me retain a healthy body fat level.

My two preferred techniques for fasting are:
1. Simply skipping breakfast results in a 15-hour period during which I do not eat. I usually eat dinner around 8:00 p.m., and instead of consuming breakfast when I wake up, I actually drink coffee and wait until around midday to eat lunch. I make it a point not to overeat at lunch. I literally eat a regular, healthy lunch. I save between 500 to 600 calories a day by skipping breakfast, and I'm able to sit in a fat-burning zone for several hours longer.

I add 60 minutes of walking at a comfortable speed throughout the morning hours to maximize the amount of fat-burning I can attain. When you haven't eaten yet, going on a short stroll is a great way to consume some extra calories.

2. I'm going on a 24-hour easy (though I continue to drink green tea or some coffee during that period). It's not as difficult as you might think to fast for a full 24 hours. People eat for a variety of reasons, including habitual actions or emotional stimuli. I've found that fasting for a whole day gives me a lot of energy and mental focus, and I can even complete a full workout regimen without eating. According to some studies, people who exercise while fasting have higher levels of growth hormone. The trick is to make sure you don't eat too much the next day. I am willing to cut a whole day's worth of calories in this manner. The idea is to restart regular, sensible eating the next day to

achieve a calorie deficit for the whole week.

Because of the Brad Pilon Eat Stop Eating scheme, I initially wanted to go on a 24-hour fast. The Eat Stop Eating website is sure to appeal to someone who wants to lose weight by following a specific diet schedule. Just a few weeks ago, Brad modified and revamped the scheme.

Fasting for weight loss is yet another way to reach your health targets. Contact me if you've skipped breakfast or been on a full-day high. When you didn't eat, what, if any, side effects did you notice? Did you lose any weight?

HOW TO LOSE WEIGHT BY INTERMITTENT FASTING?

You've just been living under a rock if you haven't heard about intermittent fasting. Intermittent fasting is without a doubt the most recent and most successful way to shed weight and keep it off indefinitely.

If you want to lose weight, eating is necessary, but fasting on occasion is also a good idea. Experts believe that prolonged fasting is an excellent way to enforce a calorie limit while also reaping the benefits of a weight-loss workout regimen.

It does not imply simply missing a meal. Intermittent fasting is described as putting the body on a fast for a period of 15 hours or more.

Bodyweight coaches believe that this is quickly becoming a common choice for people of all backgrounds who want to lose a lot of weight in a limited amount of time.

Your basal metabolic rate, or BMR for short, maybe a good indicator of how many calories you need to keep your machine going. Entering your weight, age, and height into a BMR calculator will provide a quick and accurate result. You'll get a better sense of the regular calorie needs this way. Understanding this is important because intermittent fasting must be accompanied by a food schedule that is tailored to the results. When you start eating, gorging on infinite calories will undo all of your excellent work. The best secret to a balanced weight loss diet is to fast for two days per week (not at the same time) and then follow a smart meal plan punctuated by supervised bodyweight workout routines.

If you're concerned about your energy levels or how you'll do without eating for an extended period of time, don't be concerned; just relax.

Intermittent fasting has been found in studies to increase the energy quotient whilst still fueling the metabolism, two factors that any trainer swears by for a successful performance. It's not like conventional fasting, which can leave you feeling dizzy and exhausted. In humans, fractional calorie restriction has been linked to depression and irritability. Total intermittent fasting, rather than eliminating calories from daily diet portions, will remove the complications that come with some types of fasting. This will not only boost your stamina levels but also provide you with a slew of other advantages.

Perhaps the most noticeable advantages are a reduction in high blood pressure, a reduction in diabetes, increased lifespan, reduced stress levels, and a sense of well-being, not to mention dramatic weight loss in a brief period of time.

When beginning a fasting regimen like this, begin slowly and gradually increase the length of time you fast until your body is able to tolerate a two-day fasting cycle. During this time, design appropriate bodyweight workout routines, ideally at a slow speed, before the body is capable of handling a fully-loaded exercise regimen. When you get used to it, positive changes begin to appear in your body.

If you're looking for an exercise and diet plan that can give you noticeable results in a limited amount of time, intermittent fasting is a viable choice.

I know what you're thinking: fasting? Is this going to turn out well? What are the advantages and how does it function?

All I ask is that you take a seat, unwind, and enjoy what you're about to hear. Maintain an open mind.

Intermittent fasting is a diet that follows a 16-8 fasting-to-feeding schedule. This means you can fast for 16 hours and only eat for 8 hours. Isn't it simple?

This is completely dependent on the way of life. It does not always imply that you can fast for 16 hours straight. Keep in mind that this is a lifestyle diet. It must be convenient for you. Be sure that you schedule your feedings and fastings around hours that are most convenient for you.

Don't worry if you can only fast for 16 hours for whatever reason. It's fine to end your eating window early on occasion, particularly if it's past the 8-hour mark.

So how do you start?

Before you change your diet, keep in mind that this can be a major source of discomfort for most people. It can be done in small measure. Do not expect it to be simple; it will not be. However, with the right mindset and strategy, you would undoubtedly see good results.

Often, get rid of the attitude of "Oh no, I don't get to eat until 2 p.m. today! This is going to be difficult!" It isn't going to support you. Instead, consider it a slow approach that you will implement one day at a time.

With that in mind, the 12/12 split is a good place to go.

What does the 12/12 split mean?

Simply put, the 12/12 split involves fasting for 12 hours and then eating for the next 12 hours. That is, you can fast from 7 p.m. to 7 a.m. and eat from 7 p.m. to 7 a.m. One advantage is that you won't have to make any significant changes to your eating routine. You might have to postpone breakfast or reschedule dinner, but that's it. It's very simple and convenient to put in place.

When you first start playing with the 12/12 split, you can discover that you snack in the evening. Or that you could get up in the middle of the night and force food down your throat. This is clearly an instance of feeding out of compulsion rather than hunger.

Preparing and keeping to a routine will help you become more conscious of your meal times and dietary patterns.

Tips and advice to help you get started immediately

- Begin tiny and set attainable targets for yourself. Make sure you understand what you're getting yourself into; it's all in your head, so mental planning is essential. Begin tiny and assess your progress as you go.
- Consider signing up for a free service to help you measure and monitor your current calorie intake and transition to fewer meals a day (which supports intermittent fasting).

- Keep in mind that this is a lifestyle adjustment, so it can be tailored to your preferences. Do whatever makes you more at ease.

7 REASONS WHY YOU SHOULD CONSIDER INTERMITTENT FASTING - APART FROM WEIGHT LOSS

Intermittent fasting with water can reduce your chances of developing heart disease and diabetes. The study was done in a region where up to 65 percent of the population is Mormon, who fast once a month as part of their religion.

It's interesting that this city regularly has the lowest rates of heart disease. Until recently, several experts attributed this to the Mormon Church's prohibition on smoking by its members. About the fact that the number of smokers in the United States has declined, Utah appears to have a lower incidence of heart disease than the rest of the nation.

The same study team discovered that participants who replied "yes" when asked if they fasted had less heart failure in previous studies. The new research aimed to replicate and expand on these earlier findings to see if this may be the cause for the lower incidence of heart failure.

Researchers looked at blood markers for cardiac risk in a separate report in people who hadn't eaten in the previous 12 hours. The markers were examined both when the participants were fasting and on a regular day of feeding. Participants were permitted to take medicine after the fasts, but they were only allowed to drink water.

The levels of good cholesterol (HDL) and LDL (bad) cholesterol and total cholesterol increased during the high - not ideal, to be sure, but the researchers conclude the increase was just transient. On the other hand, Fasting resulted in lower levels of unhealthy blood fats such as triglycerides and lower blood sugar levels. When you fast, the body attempts to protect its cells and tissue by relying on fats rather than sugars for energy.

Before anyone suggests fasting as a cure for heart failure, there are a couple of questions to be answered. Researchers have discovered that people who fast have a lower risk of diabetes and heart disease, but further research is needed before we can be positive.

You've already heard of juice fasts... they're all the rage on Twitter. However, comparing a water-only fast to a juice fast isn't fair. Although they can help your heart, as shown by animal tests, they are not as effective as a water-only swift.

It's also important to note that fasting isn't for everybody. This is not recommended for young children, pregnant or nursing mothers, or people with such medical conditions. If you're not sure if water quick is right for you, see the doctor. Another risk is that a fast could lead to binge eating, which would negate any health benefits you may have gained.

Although not eating will lower those percentages,

some experts believe that going to extremes is not necessarily the right option. What you eat on a daily basis has a much greater effect on the chances of heart attack than a single-day case. Often, intermittent fasting is a lifestyle option that becomes a part of your routine, not a miracle pill or silver bullet. Not only for a short time but for a long time.

Here are few other possible benefits of intermittent fasting, all of which are backed up by studies.

1. Intermittent fasting may help maintain muscle.

When you cut calories to lose weight, part of the weight you lose comes from a loss of muscle mass. This is true of both extended fasting and conventional calorie-restricted diets.

However, one study from the University of Illinois'

Department of Kinesiology and Nutrition shows that intermittent fasting could be more beneficial for maintaining muscle mass.

The researchers compared overweight and obese adults who adopted a calorie-limited diet to people of similar weight who reduced calories by fasting intermittently. The researchers discovered that both diets were similarly successful in reducing body weight and fat mass after 12 weeks, but the fasting community lost less muscle.

2. Intermittent fasting may target belly fat.

According to a study published in the journal Cell Metabolism, obese individuals who could consume whatever they wanted for 10 hours as long as they didn't eat for the other 14 hours had a decrease in waist circumference and visceral abdominal fat after 12 weeks.

3. Intermittent fasting may reduce diabetes risk.

Intermittent fasting has also been shown to reduce the risk of metabolic disorders like type 2 diabetes and heart disease, according to a study published in Cell Metabolism.

The study's participants were all diagnosed with metabolic syndrome, a group of health disorders that, when present, increase the likelihood of type 2 diabetes, stroke, and cardiac failure. These conditions include elevated blood sugar, excess abdominal fat, high blood pressure, and excessive cholesterol or triglyceride levels.

Many of the typical metabolic syndrome markers improved in all of the participants after 12 weeks.

A related analysis published in the journal Translational Research showed that alternate-day fasting resulted in clinically relevant decreases in blood sugar and insulin tolerance when participants reduced calories by 75% on a "fast day" accompanied by a "eat day" with no calorie restriction.

4. Intermittent fasting may lower high blood pressure.

According to a report published in Nutrition and Healthy after 12 weeks, people who performed 16:8 intermittent fasting without calorie counting had slightly lower systolic blood pressure than a control group.

5. Intermittent fasting could fight inflammation.

Your body's own defense against cancer, sickness, and injury is inflammation. However, there is another form of inflammation: pathological inflammation, which can cause heart disease and diabetes without being seen.

A daily diet of fatty, fried, or sugary foods and

smoking, emotional discomfort, and a regular diet of fatty, fried, or sugary foods are all general factors. Intermittent fasting has been shown in many studies to have an anti-inflammatory effect, lower the risk of metabolic disorders, and improve lung function in people with asthma.

Furthermore, according to a study published in Obesity, a decrease in inflammation caused by short-term fasting tends to shield the brain from memory disturbances and depression.

6. Intermittent fasting may reduce oxidative stress.

According to a study published in Cell Metabolism, even though you don't lose weight when fasting, your cells can profit from extra security.

Men with prediabetes were randomly allocated to either a 6-hour early eating cycle or a 12-hour feeding period, during which they could eat only from 8 a.m. until dinner around 2 p.m., fasting the rest of the day.

The men on the early time-restricted quick not only improved blood pressure and insulin sensitivity (as expected), but they also improved resistance to oxidative stress, in which unstable molecules called free radicals will destroy proteins and DNA.

7. Intermittent fasting may help you live longer. Intermittent fasting, which is much simpler to sustain than extreme calorie restriction, has also been shown to extend lifespan in rodents. In one study, rats who were allowed free access to food were found to live 83 percent longer than rats who were fed every other day.

SIDE EFFECTS OF INTERMITTENT FASTING?

While intermittent fasting can help you lose weight, it can also have a negative impact on your hormones.

This is due to the fact that body fat is the body's means of retaining energy (calories).

When you don't feed, the body goes through a series of improvements in order to make the stored energy more available.

Changes in nervous system function and significant changes in the levels of many essential hormones are examples.

Below are two metabolic changes that occur when you fast :

- **Insulin.** When you eat, your insulin levels rise, and when you fast, your insulin levels plummet. Insulin levels that are lower aid fat burning.

- **Norepinephrine (noradrenaline).** Norepinephrine is a neurotransmitter that causes fat cells to break down body fat into free fatty acids that can be burned for energy.

Interestingly, short-term fasting can increase fat burning, contrary to some advocates of eating 5–6 meals a day.

Alternate-day fasting trials of 3–12 weeks and whole-day fasting trials of 12–24 weeks have been shown to lower body weight and body fat.

Still, further research into the long-term consequences of intermittent fasting is required.

Human growth hormone (HGH) is another hormone that changes during a high, with levels rising up to five-fold.

HGH was formerly thought to aid fat burning, but recent evidence suggests it may signal the brain to save resources, making weight loss more difficult.

HGH can increase appetite and decrease energy metabolism by stimulating a limited population of agouti-related protein (AgRP) neurons.

4 INTERMITTENT FASTING SIDE EFFECTS TO WATCH OUT FOR

Intermittent fasting has grown in popularity over the past few years due to its promises of better health and weight loss. The theory is that cutting calories drastically a few times a week or limiting eating to a shorter "eating window" per day is better than cutting calories progressively at every meal, every day.

Extending fasting times (beyond the standard time between meals) stimulate cellular recovery, boost insulin sensitivity, raise levels of human growth hormone, and change gene expression in a way that improves survival and disease prevention, according to proponents. Are there, therefore, any dangers?

Before considering the risks of intermittent fasting, keep in mind that there are many types of intermittent fasting, and evidence of their long-term efficacy and protection is lacking.

The most common forms include:

- ADF fasting (alternate day fasting), which includes fasting every other day.

- Modified alternate-day fasting, in which you consumed just 25% of your normal calories the other day.

- Periodic fasting entails restricting your food intake to 500 to 600 calories per day on two days per week.

- Time-restricted diet, which restricts the "eating window" on a regular basis.

- Because some programs can have more side effects than others, it's best to talk to a doctor about the following intermittent fasting side effects before deciding on a diet that fits your lifestyle.

#1. Intermittent fasting may make you feel sick.

People can feel headaches, lethargy, crankiness, and constipation depending on how long they quick. Switching from ADFfasting to intermittent fasting or a time-restricted eating schedule that requires you to eat every day within a certain time period can help to reduce any of these unpleasant side effects.

#2. It may cause you to overeat.

Since your appetite hormones and hunger core in your brain go into overdrive while you are deprived of food, there is a definite biological push to overeat after fasting times.

"It's human nature to want to reward ourselves after performing really hard work, such as exercising or fasting for a long period of time, but there's a risk of indulging in poor eating patterns on non-fasting days."

Two typical side effects of calorie-restricted diets—slowed digestion and elevated appetite—are just as likely when people exercise intermittent fasting as when they cut calories every day, according to a

2018 report. And the evidence is mounting in studies of time-restricted eating that is out of sync with a person's circadian rhythm (their body's normal everyday pattern) will lead to metabolic issues.

#3. Intermittent fasting may cause older adults to lose too much weight.

Although intermittent fasting has shown promise, there is still less evidence regarding its benefits or how it can affect older people. Small numbers of young or middle-aged adults have been studied in humans for only brief periods of time.

However, we do know that intermittent fasting can be dangerous in some situations. "I'd be worried if you're already marginal in terms of body weight," says registered dietitian Kathy McManus, director of the Department of Nutrition at Harvard-affiliated Brigham and Women's Hospital. "Losing so much weight will damage your bones, overall immune system, and energy level."

#4. It may be dangerous if you're taking certain medications.

Dr. Eric Rimm, professor of epidemiology and nutrition at the Harvard T.H. Chan School of Public Health, advises that you can first talk to a doctor if you plan to pursue intermittent fasting. For those with such illnesses, such as diabetes, skipping meals and severely reducing calories may be harmful. Any people who take blood pressure or heart attack drugs may be more susceptible to sodium, potassium, and other mineral imbalances during longer-than-normal fasting times.

How to reduce intermittent fasting side effects

According to McManus, easing into an intermittent fasting regimen will help the body adapt. "Over a span of several months, gradually reduce the time window for feeding," she suggests.

You should also:

- Continue your medication regimen as recommended by your doctor

- Stay hydrated with calorie-free beverages, such as water and black coffee
- Choose a modified fasting plan approved by your doctor if you need to take the medication with food.

HOW LONG DOES IT TAKE FOR INTERMITTENT FASTING TO WORK?

Calorie restriction has been shown in animals to extend their lifetime and enhance their resistance to different metabolic stresses. While there is good support for calorie restriction in animal research, the evidence in human studies is not compelling. Diet supporters agree that the stress of intermittent fasting triggers an immune reaction that heals cells while still causing beneficial metabolic changes (reduction in triglycerides, LDL cholesterol, blood pressure, weight, fat mass, blood glucose). This diet's supporters are understandably concerned that they would overeat on non-fasting days and make up for calories missed while fasting. However, as opposed to other weight reduction strategies, tests have found that this is not the case.

Intermittent fasting was shown to be beneficial for weight loss in a systematic study of 40 trials, with an average loss of 7-11 pounds over 10 weeks. The experiments varied greatly in scale and length of follow-up, varying from 4 to 334 subjects and 2 to 104 weeks. It's worth noting that various research formats and intermittent fasting approaches were used, as well as participant profiles (lean vs. obese).

The fasting group was compared to a comparative group and/or a control group (either constant calorie restriction or normal lifestyle) in half of the tests, while the other half looked at an intermittent fasting group alone in the other half.

A brief summary of their findings:

- The percentage of students who dropped out varied from 0 to 65 percent. There were no major discrepancies in dropout rates between the fasting and constant calorie restriction classes. Overall, the study found that intermittent fasting did not have a low dropout rate, implying that it was not actually easier to stick to than other weight loss methods.

- There was no substantial difference in weight loss or body structure improvements in the 12 clinical trials that contrasted the fasting community to the constant calorie restriction group.

- Despite substantial weight loss and reductions in leptin hormone levels, the intermittent fasting groups did not display an overall rise in appetite in ten studies that looked at increases in appetite (a hormone that suppresses appetite).

Intermittent fasting was not shown to be more successful than daily calorie restriction in a randomized controlled study that tracked 100 obese people over a year. For the 6-month weight-loss phase, participants were assigned to either an alternating day fast (alternating days with one meal of 25% of baseline calories versus 125 percent of baseline calories divided over three meals) or daily calorie restriction (75 percent of baseline calories divided over three meals), as recommended by the American Heart Association. After 6 months, all groups' calorie levels were raised by 25% with the intention of weight maintenance. The groups' participants had common characteristics; they were mainly women and were generally well. Weight loss, compliance rates, and cardiovascular risk factors were all investigated in the study.

Their findings when comparing the two groups:

- There were no major variations in body shape, weight loss, or regain (e.g., fat mass, lean mass).

- Blood pressure, heart rate, fasting glucose, and fasting insulin did not vary significantly. Despite no discrepancies in total cholesterol or triglycerides after 12 months, the alternate-day fasting party had slightly higher LDL cholesterol levels. The writers made no mention of a potential cause.

- The alternate-day fasting party had a higher dropout rate (38%) than the daily calorie restriction community (29 percent). On non-fasting days, people in the fasting community consumed less food than recommended, but they ate more food than prescribed on fasting days.

Exactly How Much Time Does It Take For Intermittent Fasting To Work

One of the most common food patterns these days is intermittent fasting. It is very common all over the world and is recommended by people who are trying to lose weight. Reducing the feeding window to 8 hours, rather than eating regular meals during the day, is said to speed up the weight loss process by decreasing insulin levels. There are various alternatives to intermittent fasting, but they all rely on consuming a small number of calories over a brief amount of time. When it comes to intermittent fasting, the most important concern people have is how long it takes to see results.

We all know that it takes time for every diet to produce results. Intermittent fasting is the same way. According to experts, an individual must obey the simple rules for at least 10 weeks in order to see meaningful effects. If you stick to the diet for this amount of time, you should be able to lose 3 to 5 pounds (depending on your BMR).

Factors that may impact the result Getty

When practicing intermittent fasting religiously, 10 weeks is an optimal time to lose at least 3 kilograms. However, depending on one's metabolism, the outcome can vary from person to person. Weight reduction is a time-consuming operation, so effects take time to appear. So, if you're gaining weight quickly while on a diet, you're probably doing something wrong. You should re-evaluate your calorie intake right now.

Other benefits of intermittent fasting gee

Intermittent fasting not only aids weight loss but is also beneficial to mental health. According to studies, eating a low-fat, low-saturated-fat, and low-carbohydrate diet will help manage cholesterol, triglycerides, and blood sugar levels.

The diet has no side effects, but you can stick to it for a long time. However, if you have a medical problem or are pregnant, see your doctor before beginning this diet. Overall, the 16/8 approach is more long-term.

CAN I DRINK DURING INTERMITTENT FASTING?

We must first determine why we are fasting before determining what we are able to drink during intermittent fasting.

In a nutshell, there are two main causes to fast intermittently:

- Weight loss
- Health benefits

While losing weight has health benefits, most of the benefits of fasting in our bodies are due to a mechanism known as autophagy.

Low insulin levels are needed for both fat burning (ketosis) and autophagy. In light of this, a third crucial feature of intermittent fasting emerges:

- It increases insulin sensitivity,
- Improves blood sugar metabolism

- And thus fights metabolic diseases

Ketosis and Weight Loss

Fasting is essential for weight loss and it is the most efficient way to reduce insulin levels. Insulin, as a result, is the most important storage hormone in the human body.

As a result, it's in charge of telling cells to take glucose from the bloodstream and store it as fat or glycogen.

Insulin also inhibits the enzyme that breaks down body fat.

According to the report, scientists can predict about 75% of potential weight gain and loss in overweight people by studying their insulin levels.

Fasting for 16 hours cuts off the food supply, lowers insulin levels and thereby ends the body's storage mode.

After that, the body will start breaking down the carbohydrate reserves (glycogen). When the body's glycogen reserves are depleted, it will begin to burn stored fat for energy.

This fat-burning phenomenon is known as ketosis, and it is a completely normal mechanism that has guaranteed our species' longevity, contrary to popular belief.

When food is plentiful, the body is built to store fat reserves and use this fat for energy when food is scarce.

Instead of food shortages, we now have an eternal summer and snack at all hours of the day and night. As a result, we add weight.

Intermittent fasting will thus assist in reestablishing the normal equilibrium between feasting and fasting.

Insulin Resistance and Type-2-Diabetes

Intermittent fasting increases insulin sensitivity, according to science.

As a result, it lowers insulin levels, increases blood-sugar metabolism, and flushes the body of extra sugar.

It will also cure insulin resistance and type-2 diabetes, something that other diets can't do.

The liver is to blame for these metabolic disorders. Insulin resistance is a long-term effect of too much sugar and insulin in liver cells.

A fatty liver is the end product. You must burn off the deposited visceral fat in the liver if you want to get to the root of many metabolic issues.

The aggregation of fat in and near tissues, known as visceral fat, is harmful to one's health.

According to recent research intermittent eating, in

fact, will burn this unhealthy visceral fat more efficiently than low-carb diets.

On the other hand, intermittent fasting will only burn excess sugar and visceral fat if it is not broken by (liquid) food.

During intermittent fasting, it is important to avoid drinking coffee with milk because this can cause blood sugar and insulin levels to spike.

Fasting and Autophagy

For the 16 hours of intermittent fasting, autophagy is crucial. Autophagy can be induced by fasting for 14 hours.

The Nobel Prize was given for the discovery of autophagy because it is a game-changing health advantage.

When there is a scarcity of calories, the body shifts its focus from development to maintenance. As a result, autophagy, the intracellular recycling mechanism that breaks down damaged cell pieces and removes toxins from the body, is activated.

But how can be determined if a drink stops autophagy?

As a result, the human body contains three vital nutrient receptors. In a nutshell, they turn on and off the autophagy process:

- Insulin: Sensitive to carbohydrates and proteins
- mTOR: Sensitive to proteins
- AMPK: Sensitive energy shortage in cells

When energy is provided to cells – independent of macronutrients – AMP-activated protein kinase (AMPK) responds. As a result, fat, in addition to carbohydrates and proteins, inhibits autophagy.

mTOR is activated by both AMPK and insulin (mechanistic or mammalian target of rapamycin).

As a result, this growth-promoting enzyme serves

as the primary nutrient tracker, detecting nutrient supply and overriding autophagy as soon as you feed.

However, when nutrient supply is disrupted, cells react in a sustained manner, using defective cell sections for energy production.

If enabled, this intracellular recycling mechanism provides a slew of health benefits:

- Fights dementia, Alzheimer's, and Parkinson's disease
- Prevents muscle and bone atrophy
- Reduces the risk of cardiovascular disease
- Slows down aging and increases healthspan

Autophagy is the yardstick when it comes to what you should drink during intermittent fasting.

Since insulin is one of the nutrient sensors involved in autophagy, it covers all pathways that can break your fast.

Can You Drink Water During Intermittent Fasting?

Fasting is described as a period of time where you do not eat. During intermittent fasting, however, you are allowed to drink water in its purest form.

As a result, some humans can survive for over a year without fruit, but not without liquid.

Intermittent fasting also helps to deplete carbohydrate reserves, allowing the body to consume fat for energy output.

You lose a lot of water when you sprint intermittently, and your body requires water to store carbohydrates as glycogen in your liver, kidneys, and muscles.

Many that do not drink appropriately during periodic fastings can develop keto flu symptoms such as headaches or vertigo.

The shortage of minerals – especially sodium – that

your body flushes out of the water causes these minor physical ailments.

Water may supply the body with minerals in addition to the requisite fluid. Nutrient sensors, on the other hand, are not turned on in this situation. Water does not, however, crack an intermittent fast.

Furthermore, while intermittent fasting, I suggest drinking more normal Himalayan or Celtic sea salt during the feeding hours.

If you listen to your body, it will tell you that you need more salt.

Salt is beneficial because it decreases sugar cravings, enhances insulin sensitivity, boosts metabolism, and aids weight loss.

Can I Drink Carbonated Water During Intermittent Fasting?

In my opinion, carbonated water is an ideal choice when it comes to what to drink during intermittent fasting.

On the one hand, it offers effects that excellently support intermittent fasting:

- It curbs the appetite,
- Helps with an upset stomach,
- Or even with cramping.

On the other hand, Superior carbonated water can provide more than 100 mg of the necessary electrolytes magnesium, sodium, and calcium per liter to the body.

As a result, the safest choice is carbonated mineral water. But only if you can get your hands on natural, mineralized brands.

We are fortunate in Austria to have incredible

natural springs. However, depending on where you are, you can need to double-check names.

As a result, even during prolonged fasts, access to high-quality mineral water will provide electrolytes. You don't have to rely on bone broth to get them in this situation.

Can You Drink Flavored Sparkling Water While Intermittent Fasting?

While natural flavorings are now available in flavored sparkling water, most items still include sugar or sweeteners, which break the quick.

A flavoring agent that has been chemically obtained from the natural source material is known as natural flavoring.

Unless other additives are used, natural flavors can be limited to minimal amounts of macronutrients, but they have little impact on autophagy. Nonetheless, certain items are in short supply as well.

In the event of a doubt, I will not go for flavored sparkling water. Aside from that, most flavored alternatives aren't particularly tasty.

If you want to add some spice to your intermittent fasting schedule, natural flavors from fruits may be an excellent way to go.

Intermittent Fasting and Infused Water

If you want to spice your water, going the natural route is definitely the best option.

For eg, you can fill a carafe with water and a few slices of organic lime, lemon, orange, or cucumber.

This way, you will give the water a mild natural fragrance that won't interfere with your fasting if you don't eat the slices.

This assist, however, should not be used excessively. You'll be able to do without intermittent fasting until you've gotten used to it.

Can You Drink Lemon Water During Intermittent Fasting?

During intermittent fasting, a slight splash of lemon, in addition to the lemon slices, moves into the gray zone.

Let's say you want to be extra cautious. In that case, leaving a slice of organic lemon in the water is preferable, since the small quantities of calories come from carbohydrates, which can technically cause all three nutrient sensors.

On the other hand, a splash of lemon would not erase any of the effects of fasting.

Autophagy cannot be fully deactivated because there is a low baseline level of autophagy in the body at all times, particularly not by small quantities of macronutrients.

Can I Drink Coconut Water During Intermittent Fasting?

Many people claim that coconut water is an ideal intermittent fasting drink.

However, this is not the case since, unlike coconut, sugar provides the majority of the steam.

Furthermore, the electrolyte content is much smaller than one would expect – it pales in contrast to normal mineral water.

Can You Drink Tea While Intermittent Fasting?

Tea is the most common beverage on the planet, aside from wine. Tea, on the other hand, comes with a wide variety of flavors. As a result, we can't make broad generalizations and must look at each tea separately to see if it's safe to drink during a swift.

Green Tea and Intermittent Fasting

Over the years, green tea has undoubtedly proven to be the most powerful drink for intermittent fasting.

In the meantime, only coffee will challenge this title. A cup of tea contains about 2.5 calories, similar to coffee, both with (*) and without caffeine (*).

Most scholars, however, believe that the quantity of macronutrients in tea is insignificant.

Green tea, like coffee, seems to cause rather than inhibit autophagy, according to research.

In addition, all genuine tea types are suitable for intermittent fasting. The name of the tea is determined by the degree of fermentation of the tea plant "Camellia Sinensis":

- Unfermented – white tea
- Minimally fermented – Green tea
- Partially fermented – Oolong tea

- Fully fermented – black tea

Despite the fact that both of these teas are ideal for intermittent fasting, green tea has the most powerful compounds:

- Regulates blood sugar and prevents diabetes
- Boosts the metabolism
- Helps with fat burning
- Prevents cardiovascular diseases and cancer

Despite the fact that both of these teas are ideal for intermittent fasting, green tea has the best properties:

Can I Drink Herbal Tea While Intermittent Fasting?

While herbal and fruit teas are common in Central Europe, they are often a pleasant surprise. You never know what's on the inside.

Candied fruits, in addition to traditional dried fruits, are often used in fruit tea. Furthermore, they sometimes hide in herbal tea. And their sugar content can cause a fast to be broken.

As a result, there is a lot of variation in fruit tea (*). It can have almost nothing, only too much for intermittent fasting or many secret sugars, similar to green tea.

As for food transactions, the general rule is to closely read the label and prevent any questionable contents. Herbal tea, on the other hand, performs well because it does not usually contain dried fruits.

If you want to be healthy, avoid drinking herbal or fruit tea during intermittent fasting.

Ginger and Chai Tea on Intermittent Fasting

In a broad way, ginger and chai teas are similar to herbal teas in general. You should drink the brewed tea during intermittent fasting if you can find the straight dried herbs in a tea specialty store.

Please avoid instant mixes and coffee shop chai (*) because they almost always contain additives that will break yours soon.

You may be able to find straight chai (*) or ginger tea in grocery stores if you're lucky, but always read the labels before buying.

However, as most people drink chai as a latte (*), it's not easy to get it right. If it says chai latte on the bottle, you know it'll break your fast.

Ginger tea made from nothing but freshly minced ginger root and hot water, on the other hand, should be perfect as long as you don't eat the bits(*).

Can You Drink Milk During Intermittent Fasting?

It makes a difference (*) because 100 mL of milk contains not only 5 g of lactose but also about the same amount of protein.

Even a single glass of skimmed or low-fat milk will disrupt intermittent fasting by increasing blood sugar and insulin levels.

Industrially manufactured milk powder and vegetable milk drinks are not appropriate for fasting due to their composition.

Just unsweetened almond milk falls into this category. A splash in the tea after the nut milk has thinned out would not actually break the fast.

The same applies to cinnamon, which also yields exciting health benefits.

Can You Add Honey to Tea While Fasting?

Honey has a sugar content of over 80% (*). The claim that honey is pure isn't much of an advantage; table sugar is often made from "natural" beets.

Tea with sugar, as a result, is not permitted during intermittent fasting.

Tea With Sweetener

Both natural and artificial sweeteners are troublesome while fasting, as you'll see in the diet pop portion. They induce insulin even though they have no calories (Anton et al. 201018).

Tea with sweeteners is not permitted during fasting because it inhibits autophagy and fat burning.

Can You Drink Coffee During Intermittent Fasting?

While coffee is often prohibited for religious reasons, it does not usually interfere with intermittent fasting.

Coffee, on the other hand, does not suppress but also stimulates autophagy.

As a result, researchers have discovered that both caffeinated and decaffeinated coffee can cause autophagy in muscles, the liver, the heart, and other essential organs.

While coffee itself does not break a fast, additives such as sugar do.

- Milk and skimmed milk
- Cream and creamer
- Soy and oat milk
- Sweeteners

And with a splash of almond milk, you would be able to get away with it. Even the thin nut milk, though, practically breaks the quick.

More information can be found in my comprehensive guide to coffee and intermittent fasting:

Black Coffee and Espresso
A cup of black coffee can contain 1-4 calories as well as trace amounts of protein, fat, and other nutrients.

As a result, the nutrients in 1-2 cups of black coffee are insufficient for most people to affect their metabolism in a way that will enable them to break their fast (van Dam et al. 200420).

Since caffeine can help reduce hunger, many people are able to fast for longer periods of time.

Significant amounts of caffeine can affect intermittent fasting by stimulating the hormone adrenaline, which strengthens our bodies for stressful conditions.

As a result, glucose will reach the bloodstream without the need for calories.

Coffee would not prevent autophagy in this indirect manner if you don't drink more than 1-2 cups in a short amount of time.

You should drink a cup of coffee at a time during intermittent fasting due to the following properties:

- Rich in antioxidants, which curb the appetite
- Induces and supports autophagy
- Increases metabolic rate
- Supports sustainable weight loss

As a result, espresso or black coffee is a great drink to have when your appetite returns. However, it would be beneficial if you did not drink a large amount of it.

Can You Drink Bulletproof Coffee During Intermittent Fasting?

Bulletproof Coffee is not suitable for fasting, despite claims to the contrary.

While keto coffee does not raise insulin levels, it does provide a significant amount of fat to the body.

And, as we all know, fat activates the nutrient sensor AMPK. As a result, Bulletproof Coffee has an impact on autophagy.

Bulletproof Coffee does not raise insulin levels because it contains only pure, high-quality fat and no other macronutrients.

As a result, you'll be able to remain in ketosis and burn fat.

This coffee with MCT oil and butter lets beginners get used to intermittent fasting because it suppresses hunger.

If you can only fast for 12 hours on black coffee but 18 hours on a few teaspoons of coconut oil, the fat addition is possibly justified.

After a few days of 16/8 intermittent fasting,

though, you won't need these training wheels to keep the fast going.

Eventually, you'll want to burn body fat rather than muscle.

Can I Drink Bone Broth During Intermittent Fasting?

Bone broth made from beef, pork, or chicken bones is not only delicious, but it also has properties that aid fasting:

- It Supplies electrolytes
- Is easily digestible
- Contains natural fat that helps to absorb nutrients

But here's the thing: broth has enough fat in it to trigger AMPK and crack a high.

As a result, bone broth is the best option for breaking a short.

Since bone broth is high in magnesium, potassium,

calcium, and sodium, it may help to replenish electrolytes that have been washed away.

As a result, bone broth can be used as an electrolyte source during fasting, such as during days or weeks of fasting. As a result, it's better used as a set of training wheels for intermittent fasting.

Can I Drink Pickle Juice While Intermittent Fasting?

The water of sugar-free pickles, including bone broth, has aided many people during fasting. Although the bone broth is an electrolyte powerhouse, the cucumber water adds salt in particular.

If you have physical discomfort, such as a headache, you should drink it during sporadic or extended fasting.

Cucumber water, on the other hand, can be used for this same purpose.

Can You Drink Apple Cider Vinegar During Intermittent Fasting?

Apple cider vinegar boosts nutrient digestion, making it easier to ingest healthier fats and incorporate them into one's diet.

Drinking apple vinegar also helps with intermittent fasting because of the following effects:

- Reduces blood sugar and promotes insulin sensitivity
- Increases satiety and reduces the risk of overeating
- Stimulates fat burning and helps lose weight
- Releases stomach and intestinal neutralizing hormones and ions
- Works against heartburn and acid reflux

For these causes, apple cider vinegar is revered by advocates of low-carb diets such as the keto diet.

In addition, apple cider vinegar mixed with water is commonly used by fasting beginners. An apple cider vinegar drink could affect autophagy from a strictly technological standpoint, but the tiny amounts of macronutrients in most cases are negligible (*).

Nonetheless, it is an assist for new fasting distances, similar to broth, and its properties make it a first-class drink for breaking a fast.

Can You Drink Juice While Intermittent Fasting?

Juices are sometimes referred to as "natural things." Is it, though, possible to consume them while fasting intermittently?

Fasting, Fruit and Vegetable Juice

Juice intake is much more detrimental to one's health than eating whole foods.

Juice causes massive blood sugar and insulin surges when the antioxidant fiber is removed from the skin.

The fructose in fruit juices often explodes through the liver uncontrolled, inducing insulin resistance and visceral fat in the long term, precisely since the antioxidant influence of dietary fibers is absent.

As a result, non-alcoholic fatty liver (NAFL) is much more common than alcoholic fatty liver disease.

Fruit juice not only breaks the hard, but it's no better than a coke – no matter how "organic." Anyone who is adamant about losing weight must keep their hands off it at all times, including at mealtimes.

Can You Drink Celery Juice While Intermittent Fasting?

Even though celery is on my low-carb food list, juicing makes it a lunch.

The quick is broken because neither celery juice nor other vegetable juices are calorie-free. Furthermore, sugar is the primary source of energy in celery and is what causes insulin to be stimulated.

Can You Drink Smoothies During Intermittent Fasting?

Since smoothies are mixed rather than juiced, they have some fiber, but they split an intermittent fast.

They are the lesser of two evils in comparison to fruit juices, but they also count as a meal.

But Can You Drink Lemonade While Fasting?

Lemonade cannot be consumed during intermittent fasting because it contains sugar. As a result, to be permitted during intermittent fasting, you'd have to limit it to lemon water.

But what if the lemonade were sweetened with zero-calorie sweeteners rather than sugar?

Can You Drink Diet Soda While Intermittent Fasting?

When it comes to intermittent fasting, the sweet taste is a hot subject. On the one hand, getting rid of it is still difficult. On the other side, it also encourages cravings.

Proteins, starch, fat, and calories are also absent from most sugar-free sweeteners.

However, several diet gurus overlook the fact that blood sugar alone does not cause insulin release.

On the other hand, Sweeteners have the potential to raise insulin levels even higher than sugar in standard coke.

Fasting and Diet Coke

Aspartame, which has been the basis for diet coke for decades, is one of the most well-known sweeteners.

While aspartame has little effect on blood sugar levels, it does raise insulin levels faster than table sugar (Anton et al. 201032).

As a result, the sweetener in diet coke inhibits both autophagy and fat burning.

With this in mind, it's certainly no coincidence that people who drink many diet drinks are usually considerably overweight.

Intermittent Fasting and Coke Zero

While the ingredients in Cola Zero vary, it often contains aspartame and acesulfame K.

According to research, the heat-stable sweetener acesulfame-K used in zero beverages raises insulin levels to the same amount as glucose.

As a result, coke zero is ineffective for weight loss and autophagy.

Furthermore, zero-calorie sweeteners cause brain

cravings, which is not compatible with intermittent fasting.

As a result, researchers discovered that substituting zero and light drinks for normal soft drinks does not result in the required calorie loss due to increased appetite.

Green Coke and Stevia

Advertisements promote stevia as the best natural sweetener. Nonetheless, it is harvested from a plant and processed by chemical methods, much as table sugar from sugar beet.

With this in mind, the sweetener in Green Cola doesn't seem so natural.

Furthermore, the plant-based sweetener has the following drawbacks:

- Increases insulin levels
- Alters the gut microbiome

So here we are in a precise condition. Intermittent fasting is not compatible with stevia or green cola.

Will You Drink Energy Drinks While You're on an Intermittent Fasting Diet?

Sugar is present in most energy drinks. As a result, you can't drink them while you're fasting intermittently.

Zero Calorie Energy Drinks

Red Bull Sugarfree, like coke zero, contains aspartame and acesulfame K.

Fasting is not possible for sugar-free energy drinks because they use chemical sweeteners.

Intermittent Fasting Energy and Amino Acid Drinks

What are branched-chain amino acids (BCAAs) and why are they used in sports drinks? Expansion!

As a result, they activate the human body's primary (muscle) development pathway, mTOR.

As a result, drinking Bang Energy or other amino acid beverages stops the body from fasting and allows it to rise.

As previously said, mTOR is our bodies' primary nutrient sensor, which inhibits autophagy. In brief, anti-fasting liquids like Bang Energy and other amino acid drinks can be avoided during intermittent fasting.

Gatorade and Powerade Zero While Intermittent Fasting

Even if the addition of electrolytes and vitamins

sounds appealing for fasting, sugar-free sports drinks are not recommended.

Sucralose, the sweetener in Splenda, is used in Gatorade and Powerade Zero, for example.

According to research, only one pack of Splenda will wipe out half of the balanced gut flora.

Sucralose also raises insulin levels by around 20%, which breaks fasting in any case.

Protein Shakes and Intermittent Fasting

Scientists didn't realize that protein even activates insulin until the 1990s.

As a result, the first low-carb diets, such as the Atkins diet, failed miserably. The keto diet's current success can be attributed to the fact that it is founded on this very recent experience.

Protein shakes, on the other hand, also have the

reputation of being a weight-loss beverage. A protein shake of separated whey protein, on the other hand, is unlikely to activate insulin and the primary nutrient sensor mTOR.

Protein Shakes not only crack a fast, but they also suppress autophagy, a process that helps to minimize unhealthy protein accumulations, such as those in the brain.

As a result, autophagy protects us from modern diseases characterized by excessive protein and development, such as dementia, cardiovascular disease, and cancer.

Can You Drink Alcohol While Intermittent Fasting?

Alcohol can not be consumed during intermittent fasting because the effects are worse on an empty stomach.

Furthermore, alcohol is a calorie-dense beverage that, by definition, breaks a fast.

It's still not a good idea to drink alcohol at mealtimes. Cocktails, mixed drinks, and especially beer are high in carbohydrates, which stimulate insulin and hunger.

Red wine is an exception and can be consumed in a bottle with dinner. Red wine has a beneficial effect on blood sugar, cholesterol, and insulin levels when consumed with food.

A dry red wine, such as Pinot Noir, can help to increase insulin sensitivity.

What You Can Drink During Intermittent Fasting!

If you don't want to read the rest of this page, you can skip ahead to the following section: The bottom line is as follows:

This is a list of beverages that should be consumed during intermittent fasting, according to science:

- Water
- Mineral Water
- Infused water with slices of lemon, orange, or cucumber
- Lemon water no additives
- Black coffee no additive
- Black decaffeinated coffee
- White tea no additives
- Green tea
- Oolong tea
- Black tea
- Herbal tea no sweeteners
- Diluted apple cider vinegar (auxiliary agent)

What you will drink during an intermittent fasting period is only determined by your objectives. If your main target is to lose weight, stick to the suggestions above.

When it comes to long-term fasting for anti-aging and disease prevention, scholars and experts have differing viewpoints.

Despite the fact that several animal experiments show that coffee and green tea promote autophagy, we don't know for sure.

Since there is no evidence of autophagy in humans, many people limit autophagy fasting to plain water fasting, with only salt or mineral water added if required.

Green tea, on the other hand, activated autophagy in human cells, which had previously been injected into mice.

HOW MUCH WEIGHT CAN YOU LOSE IN A MONTH WITH INTERMITTENT FASTING?

There are many different ways to lose weight.

Intermittent fasting is a technique that has gained popularity in recent years.

Daily, short-term fasts — or times of little or no food intake — are part of an eating trend known as intermittent fasting.

Intermittent fasting is commonly thought of as a weight-loss strategy. People who fast for brief periods of time consume fewer calories, which can lead to weight loss over time.

On the other hand, intermittent fasting can help reduce diabetes and cardiovascular disease risk factors by lowering cholesterol and blood sugar levels.

Choosing your intermittent fasting plan

Intermittent fasting can be done in a variety of ways. Among the most common are:

- the 16:8 method
- the 5:2 diet
- the Warrior diet
- Eat Stop Eat
- alternate-day fasting (ADF)

Both strategies can be useful, but determining which one works better for you is a personal decision.

Here's a rundown of the benefits and drawbacks of each approach to help you decide which is best for you.

The 16/8 method

One of the most common fasting plans for weight loss is the 16/8 intermittent fasting method.

Food and calorie-containing drinks are limited to an 8-hour window a day under the package. It necessitates fasting for the remaining 16 hours of the day.

While other diets have rigid guidelines and regulations, the 16/8 approach is more versatile and is based on a time-restricted feeding (TRF) model.

You can eat calories during every 8 hours.

Few people stop eating late and keep to a 9 a.m. to 5 p.m. schedule, while others miss breakfast and fast from noon to 8 p.m.

Limiting the number of hours you may eat during the day can aid in weight loss and blood pressure reduction.

According to research, time-restricted eating habits, such as the 16/8 cycle, can help avoid hypertension and decrease food consumption, resulting in weight loss.

The 16/8 form, when paired with strength exercise, helped male participants lose weight and retain muscle mass, according to a 2016 report.

More recent research discovered that the 16/8 approach had little effect on muscle or power increases in women doing resistance exercises.

Although the 16/8 approach can be quickly incorporated into any lifestyle, some people may find it difficult to go 16 hours without food.

Furthermore, consuming too many chips or unhealthy food during the 8-hour fasting time will counteract the benefits of 16/8 intermittent fasting.

To reap the most nutritional benefits from this diet, consume a well-balanced diet rich in fruits, vegetables, whole grains, healthy fats, and protein.

The 5:2 method

The 5:2 diet is a simple intermittent fasting strategy.

You eat regularly five days a week and don't count

calories. Then you cut your calorie consumption to one-quarter of your standard requirements on the remaining two days of the week.

For someone who eats 2,000 calories a day on a daily basis, this will include cutting their calorie consumption to 500 calories two days a week.

According to a 2018 report, the 5:2 diet is almost as good for weight loss and blood glucose management in people with type 2 diabetes as daily calorie restriction.

Another research showed that the 5:2 diet was almost as good for weight loss and the treatment of metabolic disorders like heart disease and diabetes as constant calorie restriction.

The 5:2 diet allows you to choose which days you fast, and there are no restrictions on whether or what you eat on full-calorie days.

It's worth noting, though, that eating "normally" on full-calorie days does not imply that you can consume anything you want.

And if it's only for two days a week, limiting yourself to 500 calories a day is difficult. Furthermore, eating too few calories can cause you to become ill or faint.

While the 5:2 diet can be beneficial, it is not for all. Consult a physician to see if the 5:2 diet is right for you.

Eat Stop Eat

Brad Pilon, author of the book "Eat Stop Eat," popularized an unorthodox approach to intermittent fasting called "Eat Stop Eat."

This intermittent fasting schedule entails deciding on one or two non-consecutive days a week that you can go without food for a 24-hour cycle.

You can eat as much as you like the rest of the week, so it's best to eat a well-balanced diet to stop overindulging.

A weekly 24-hour fast is justified by the belief that eating fewer calories would result in weight loss.

Fasting for up to 24 hours will induce a metabolic change, causing the body to use fat instead of glucose as an energy source.

However, abstaining from food for 24 hours at a time takes a lot of effort, which can contribute to bingeing and overeating afterward. It may also result in disordered eating habits.

Further research is required to ascertain the Eat Stop Eat diet's possible health benefits and weight loss properties.

Before you try Eat Stop Eat, talk to the doctor to see if it's a good weight-loss plan for you.

Alternate-day fasting

Alternate-day fasting is a simple, easy-to-follow intermittent fasting plan. You fast every single day on this diet, so you can eat anything you want on the non-fasting days.

On fasting days, some variations of this diet follow an "updated" fasting approach that includes consuming about 500 calories. Some models, on the other hand, fully exclude calories on fasting days.

Alternate-day fasting has proven weight loss benefits.

In a randomized pilot trial of adults with obesity, alternate-day fasting was found to be as beneficial for weight loss as everyday calorie restriction.

Another study showed that after transitioning between 36 hours of fasting and 12 hours of unlimited feeding for four weeks, participants ate 35% fewer calories and lost an average of 7.7 pounds (3.5 kg) (12).

If you're serious about losing weight, incorporating a workout routine into your daily routine will help.

According to research, mixing alternate-day fasting with endurance training will result in weight loss that is twice as effective as simply fasting.

Fasting for a full day any other day can be challenging, particularly if you're new to the practice. On non-fasting days, it's easy to go overboard.

If you're new to intermittent fasting, start with a changed fasting schedule to ease into alternate-day fasting.

It's better to eat a healthy diet, including high protein foods and low-calorie vegetables, to make you feel whole, whether you begin with a modified fasting schedule or a complete quick.

The Warrior diet

The Warrior Diet is a fasting regimen based on the dietary patterns of ancient warriors.

Ori Hofmekler created the Warrior Diet in 2001, which is stricter than the 16:8 solution but less so than the Eat Fast Eat process.

It entails eating very little during the day for 20 hours and then eating as much as needed during a 4-hour time at night.

During the 20-hour fast, the Warrior Diet allows dieters to eat limited quantities of dairy ingredients, hard-boiled eggs, fresh fruits, and vegetables, as well as non-calorie beverages.

After a 20-hour fast, people have a 4-hour window to eat whatever they want, as long as it's unprocessed, nutritious, and/or organic.

Although no study has been done on the Warrior Diet directly, human trials have shown that time-restricted eating periods can help people lose weight.

Other health benefits of time-restricted feeding periods are unknown. In mice, time-restricted feeding cycles have been shown to inhibit diabetes, slow tumor growth, postpone aging, and extend lifespan.

More analysis on the Warrior Diet is required to comprehend its weight-loss advantages truly.

The Warrior Diet can be impossible to stick to because it limits calorie intake to just 4 hours a day. Overeating late at night is a common issue.

The Warrior Diet has been linked to eating disorders. If you're up for the challenge, see a physician and see if it's right for you.

INTERMITTENT FASTING AND THE PHASE 1 DIET FOR MAXIMUM FAT BURNING

It's possible that certain readers are only familiar with one or the other. Both have a distinct style that helps with weight reduction and overall fitness. Just one of them seems to be a "diet" on the floor, but even the word is used loosely. I am very familiar with all of them in terms of weight reduction and general health benefits, so I can have an overview of both. I sincerely feel that by bridging the difference and combining these two approaches, you will be able to achieve some truly remarkable weight loss outcomes. Let's get started!

Fasting For Fat Loss Is Extremely Effective

The notion of fasting as part of a meal schedule is mostly met with scorn in the health community. Many businesses and coaches convince us that if we don't feed every few hours, our metabolisms will slow down and our bodies will go into "starvation mode." Before we go any further, let's determine that "slowing the metabolism" is perhaps one of the main fitness industry theories. Chronic, low-calorie intake that lasts weeks results in a reduction in metabolism. When you fast a couple of days a week, this does not happen.

Here's a quick rundown on how intermittent fasting can be incorporated into someone's daily routine. I'll explain how this can be tweaked to your liking later.

1. Normally eat until dinner (2-4 meals, not 6-8)

2. Eat your dinner but stop eating after that.

3. Fast until dinner the following day. (No calorie consumption)

4. For that meal just eat a regular size dinner.

You're still fasting for 24 hours, so you're eating a meal every day with this method. This is usually performed once or twice a week. You should fast three days a week if you need to lose a lot of weight before a holiday or reunion. This is something I will only do for a few weeks.

What You Learn About Yourself During Fasting

You should keep track of any changes in your eating habits when fasting. After a few attempts at a 24-hour short, the explanations for what, where, and why you eat can become clear. We feed for a variety of reasons, like emotional ties or sheer instinct, rather than hunger. We are often so programmed to feed at specific hours that we eat when we aren't hungry.

Intermittent Fasting Is A Lifestyle And Not A Diet

It is not classified as a "diet" and does not limit you to certain ingredients, meals, mixes, guidelines, or maps to lose weight. It encourages you to break free from compulsive eating habits and enjoy more flexibility in your diet. Adding a range of foods to your diet will deter you from overeating some kind of "evil" food, rather than totally eliminating it because someone ordered you to. Let's move on to a more in-depth discussion of diet and health now that we've developed this field of weight loss.

What Is The Phase One Diet AKA The Fungus Link?

Doug Kaufmann is the brains behind the theory that fungi and yeast play a role in poor health and inability to lose weight. He has studied and recorded how fungi create toxic compounds known as "mycotoxins," which are responsible for a variety of health issues. He not only addresses the issue by treating places where spores and yeast will invade the body, but he also offers a cure by starving the disease and thereby reversing the effects of so many of America's health issues. He discovered that fungi, like humans, had a craving for particular carbohydrates. The Phase 1 Diet is simple to follow once you realize that fungi require carbohydrates to survive inside the body.

So What Is Allowed On The Phase 1 Diet?

This is the only "diet" I would ever suggest that bans specific foods, but only for a specific reason. Excluding some ingredients for a short period of time starves and kills the parasite while still revealing the source of food cravings. Uncontrollable food cravings can be harmful to your fitness, as can the extra pounds on your belly, legs, hips, and other body parts. Fungus overgrowth could be the cause of weight loss failure. You will have to eat mindlessly as long as you are hooked to those foods. Many people's fitness improves to the point that they can't believe how good they do. The unique food preference that starves and avoids fungus overgrowth is one of the main reasons for this. This revolutionary approach to food has improved the lives of many people.

Here's a brief rundown on what foods are allowed on the Phase 1 Diet.

Example of Acceptable Foods For The Phase 1 Diet

1)Eggs

2)FRUIT: Green Apples, Avocado, Coconut, Berries, Lemon, Lime,

3)MEATS

4)VEGETABLES: Fresh, unblemished vegetables and freshly made vegetable juice

5)BEVERAGES: Bottled or filtered water, freshly squeezed carrot juice, non-sweeteners additives water.

6) VINEGAR: apple cider vinegar

7) OILS: olive, grape, flaxseed, cold-pressed virgin coconut oil

8) NUTS: raw nuts, Stored nuts tend to gather mold.

9) SWEETENERS: Stevia, Xylitol

10) DAIRY: Organic Butter, Organic Yogurt, unsweetened whipping cream and real sour cream.

Note: Once again, these food options are only permitted at the start of the diet. After a while, you will incorporate more and more food types, but only after the fungus overgrowth has been addressed. There are a few steps that he has set up so that you aren't left wondering what to do next. Remember the diet restrictions are only in place for a limited time. I sincerely agree that combining this diet with intermittent fasting would eliminate all of the guesswork from weight loss. Losing weight is just a matter of eating more calories than you consume. Intermittent starvation causes a large calorie deficiency, whereas the Phase 1 Diet breaks dietary addictions that lead to obesity and fungus-related health issues.

PROOF THAT INTERMITTENT FASTING AND BODYBUILDING WORK TOGETHER

With intermittent fasting becoming more common as a weight-loss and health-management diet, it's vital to know how to get started. Here are three tips to help you get started with intermittent fasting as soon as possible.

- Intermittent fasting doesn't have to be a quick fix for weight loss; in fact, it's much more effective as a real lifestyle option. As a result, the first decision to make is how to adjust to YOUR life quickly. Remember that depending on what you're trying to do, the fast will last anywhere from 16 hours to multiple days. An alternating day (24-hour) fast/eat cycle or a 16/8 cycle are the two methods that are possibly the simplest to set up.

- When should I go to the gym? This is a crucial question. Diet is without a doubt the most crucial factor in weight loss and healthy health, so the re-feed can align with your exercise to get the most out of an occasional easy. Personally, I've had decent results with a quick from 8 p.m. to lunch the next day and an early afternoon workout. All of the food I consume around my exercise is used for nutrition and muscle recovery rather than being stored as body fat.

- What am I hoping to do by fasting intermittently? Is your goal to lose weight, add muscle, or enhance your fitness, or a combination of the three? You will begin to determine how long your fast should be and how much food you can consume during the eating "window" based on your answers to these questions.

Proof That Intermittent Fasting and Bodybuilding Work Together

Sergio Nubret, one of the most well-known bodybuilders of his time, was a proponent of intermittent fasting even before it became fashionable. Sergio Nubret had a great physique, and the question is not whether he designed it with steroids or not, but rather what his culinary practices were.

Amazing Body

Sergio Nubret was well-known not only for his incredible physique but also for his eating habits. In the African bush, he ate like a lion. He didn't go about chasing antelope and zebra. He only ate one massive meal a day and fasted for the rest of the day. Intermittent fasting was essentially what he was doing. He had a window in which he would enjoy his lunch and another in which he would not.

Can you emulate him using intermittent fasting?

Sergio Nubret was well-known for both his physique and his eating habits. In the African bush, he gorged himself like a lion. He didn't go chasing zebras and antelopes. Per day, he ate only one massive meal and fasted the rest of the time. Intermittent fasting is essentially what he was doing. He had a slot that he would feed and another where he would not.

Calorie Surplus for muscle building

At the end of the day, whether or not you should develop strength comes down to whether or not you're in a calorie surplus. If you're exercising slowly and are in a calorie surplus, you'll gain muscle, which means intermittent fasting and bodybuilding can be beneficial to you. Sergio Nubret found it to be successful, and he only ate one meal a day. Brad Pilon, John Berardi, Martin Berkhan, and the Hodgetwins are only a few of the many people who have seen substantial muscle growth during intermittent fasting.

What works for you?

As for something, it may or may not be the right solution for you; the main thing is to figure out why it is the case and not to ignore anything until you have given it a try. Intermittent fasting has many advantages, and when paired with a good fitness regimen and adequate diet, you will develop muscle to bodybuilding levels. Give it a go and let me know how it goes.

MY EXPERIENCE WITH INTERMITTENT FASTING

Intermittent fasting may seem to be a dangerous way to lose weight by starving the body, but this is not the case. It is intermittent starvation, not daily starvation, as the name suggests because the routine is beneficial rather than harmful. It does not necessitate erratic eating, but just the opposite. This means that a person can continue to eat as they usually do without worrying about their calorie intake. So, since breakfast consists of bacon and eggs, lunch consists of a subway sandwich, and dinner consists of lasagna, this eating routine does not need to be broken. The only distinction would be a 24-hour pause during which the only thing to be eaten will be water. This swift is essentially a break from fats, sugars, and proteins for the digestive system. The idea is to rest the internal system rather than overworking it as a result of excessive food intake and less time to burn it off by aerobic and anaerobic activities. The greatest part of this "break" is that the body slows up and any impurities are flushed out at this period when water is the only substance consumed.

In reality, it is not the hunger of a day that produces the desired effects but rather the water intake. The benefits of water have been recorded since the dawn of time. The doctor emphasizes the importance of drinking plenty of water with any ailment. Water is essential for keeping acne at bay and maintaining a healthy glow, according to beauticians. Dieticians emphasize the importance of drinking plenty of water. Even for aerobic and anaerobic activities, the importance of drinking plenty of water is repeatedly emphasized. So, what kind of spell does water cast on the body to make it such a dependable agent?

Water, as previously said, accelerates the body's metabolism. Since the kidneys need water to work correctly, and most people consume insufficient amounts of water, it is up to the liver to compensate for the water lost. This reduces the liver's overall production or efficiency. Since one of the key roles of the liver is to metabolize the fat that has been processed, since performing the tasks for the kidney, the liver is unable to metabolize the fat, resulting in a rise in the number of additional pounds that have been added to the amount.

A day dedicated to a 24-hour irregular fast, which can last up to 36 hours depending on the person's will, is a day dedicated. As a result, the body concentrates more on the accumulated fats and effectively burns them off. So the no-food day is mainly a day to rev up the metabolism in order to burn out all of the excess fat that the body has accumulated as a result of not consuming enough water.

Apart from speeding up the metabolism, another benefit of intermittent fasting for the body is that it aids in the loss of all water weight accumulated in the body. The main reason for the water storage in the hips, calves, knees, and stomach is due to an irregular water flow. The body retained all the water because it was not consuming the necessary amount every day. As a result, once the water intake is abundant, the body chooses to release all of the water contained in the form of fat and greatly reduces body weight.

Furthermore, it has been found that when enough water is consumed, the body needs fewer calories. As a result, during the intermittent fasting period, when the body drinks a large amount of water, there is less of a need for food, so the stomach continues to be well-nourished. Water also aids in the preservation of muscle mass, allowing for more effective workouts. So, whether you want to go for a 45-minute walk or get up on the treadmill during your sporadic easy, staying hydrated is the secret to feeling good right after the workout.

Intermittent fasting is, without a doubt, the most effective way to maintain a stable weight loss regimen. On the other hand, the outcomes will not be instantaneous, but there will not be a week where a 1lb reduction does not turn up on the scale. Adopting this ritual is a smart strategy for losing weight.

My Experience With Intermittent Fasting the 5:2 Way

Past Eating

For the past 4-5 years, I've been through a variety of eating types. I was on the Wheat Belly diet, then Keto, and then my thyroid went out of whack, something I now refer to the Keto (low carb) diet, and I've since heard of a lot of people who have seen the same thing with decreased carbohydrates.

During my recovery from hyperthyroidism, I ate everything and all, and there was a stretch of time when I encouraged myself to eat whatever I wanted, whenever I wanted, and there was a lot of healing over body shame and embarrassment overeating. It looked like a pendulum had swung out from such a restrictive diet.

Then I discovered the Medical Medium, and my health began to improve dramatically. During that time, I stopped eating meat and chicken and went vegan 90% of the time, with the exception of eggs and fish, which I couldn't do without.

5:2 Intermittent Fasting
I've been adopting the 5:2 Diet for the past month. I choose not to refer to it as a diet because it is more like a way of life. Michael Mosley, a British writer, was the first to popularize it. I was hooked after watching his documentary.

Anything revolves around Intermittent Fasting. There are many forms of intermittent fasting, but the 5:2 Diet involves regularly eating for five days a week and fasting for two days a week (based on a quarter of the daily calorie allowance). Many people find this way of eating to be more manageable than traditional calorie-restricted diets.

Health Benefits and Weight Loss
I've long given up on weight loss as a goal; if it

happens, great, but the health benefits of eating this way have been well established. I'm particularly interested in seeing how it affects my high blood pressure.

Many people have shed weight and improved their metabolic fitness by eating this way. When the body isn't still digesting, it has the time to heal and regenerate.

One of the things I liked about this way of eating is that it deceives your body into thinking it isn't being deprived, causing it to go into hunger mode and store fat. I've never been able to lose weight on other diets because of this.

Low Carb But Not Keto

I've figured out what my body prefers to eat on these two days, which has helped the transition go more smoothly. I've discovered foods that satisfy my hunger while being low in calories. And I'm not on a Keto diet; instead, I'm going for a Whole Food Plant-Based Diet. It was difficult at first, but by tweaking my meals, I was able to make it simpler.

What Days To Fast

I was fasting Tuesday and Saturday, but I realized I needed to change it because I had a PT session on Friday and needed more food to heal on Saturday. As a result, I've switched to Monday and Thursday.

Non-Fast Days

I was fasting Tuesday and Saturday but realized I wanted to change it because I had a PT session on Friday and needed more food to heal on Saturday.

As a result, Monday and Thursday have been added to my schedule.

Support

I'm a member of a Facebook community for this diet, and a lot of people say they can go all day without eating and then consume all of their calories at dinner, but I can't. I feel so irritable. lol, I have to eat three meals a day, so I've figured out how to do that. The groups are a wonderful source of encouragement, and you will get food suggestions from them. I recently purchased three books on this way of eating, two of which are vegetarian.

To keep track of my calories, I use the myfitnesspal app. When I'm at the grocery, I use the bar code scanner to determine the calorie content of various items. I'd never measured calories before, so this was a new experience for me.

It's still early days for me, so I'll keep you updated on my progress.

(If you're thinking of trying this way of eating, talk to a doctor first; it's not approved for pregnant or breastfeeding mothers, people with diabetes, or people who have eating disorders.)

FREQUENTLY ASKED QUESTIONS, CONCERNS, AND COMPLAINTS

I'm a woman. Should I do anything differently?

I haven't consulted with women to help them follow an intermittent fasting regimen, so I can't comment on this.

However, I've learned that when doing regular intermittent fasting, women can find a broader window of eating to be more beneficial. Women can achieve better results by eating for 10 hours and fasting for 14 hours instead of men, who typically fast for 16 hours and then eat for 8 hours. Experiment to see what works best for you, not just for women, is the best advice I can offer anybody. Your body will send you messages. Pay attention to what the body likes.

If you're a woman, there's even an all-female Facebook page dedicated to intermittent fasting. I'm sure you'll find a wealth of useful information and resources there.

I could never skip breakfast. How do you do it?
I don't think so. Breakfast foods are my favorites, so I eat them every day at 1 p.m.

Also, I think you'll be shocked by how much stamina you have in the morning if you eat a huge dinner the night before. The majority of people's fears or doubts about intermittent fasting stem from the fact that their employers have told them that they need to eat breakfast or eat every three hours, and so on. My own experiences do not affirm it, and neither does science.

I thought you were supposed to eat every 3 hours?
You may have read that you should consume six meals a day, or that you should eat every three hours, or something similar.

Here's why this was a common concept for a short

time:

When the body is cooking food, it burns calories. The theory behind the more meals plan was that you would lose more calories if you fed more often during the day. As a result, taking more meals can aid in weight loss.

Here's the problem:

The size of the food your body is processing determines how many calories you burn. As a result, digesting six smaller meals totaling 2000 calories expends the same amount of energy as processing two big meals totaling 1000 calories.

You'll end up in the same spot if you consume your calories in ten meals or one.

This is crazy. If I didn't eat for 24 hours, I'd die.

To be honest, I believe the mental barrier is the most significant factor preventing people from fasting, as it is not difficult to do in reality.

Here are a few reasons why intermittent fasting isn't as ridiculous as you would imagine.

For starters, different religious sects have practiced fasting for decades. For thousands of years, medical professionals have recognized the health effects of fasting. Fasting, in other words, isn't a passing fad or a clever publicity trick. It's been around for a long time and has proven to be successful.

Second, many of us are unfamiliar with fasting because it is hardly discussed. The explanation for this is that convincing you not to eat their products, take their vitamins, or purchase their merchandise would not give them any money. Fasting, in other words, isn't a particularly marketable subject, so you don't see any advertisement or promotion about it.

As a consequence, it seems intense or odd, despite the fact that it is not.

Third, even though you don't realize it, you've actually already fasted many days. Have you ever had a late brunch since sleeping in late on the weekends? This is something that some people do every weekend. Under these cases, we always skip dinner the night before and often wait until 11 a.m., noon, or much longer to eat. You didn't even realize you were fasting for 16 hours.

Finally, even though you don't intend on doing intermittent fasting regularly, I recommend doing one 24-hour fast. It's a smart idea to teach yourself that you can go a day without eating. Fasting also has a number of health advantages, which I've shown in this book through numerous scientific trials.

CONCLUSION

Fasting used to be synonymous with religious or philosophical practices and rituals. However, an increasing number of fitness fans are starting to incorporate intermittent fasting into their lives as a way to reduce weight and boost physical health and lifespan, based on their goals and circumstances.

From an evolutionary standpoint, intermittent fasting (IF) makes complete sense. The meat was either plentiful or exceedingly sparse for our paleolithic forefathers on a daily basis. As a result, we progressed during periods of dietary restriction.

When there is a lack of resources, the body activates "repair and care" genes. These genes boost the development of essential chemicals including glutathione, which aids in the repair of tissues that would otherwise go unrepaired during periods of abundance. Cells will survive longer as a result of this adaptation.

Intermittent fasting is described as a time of fasting followed by a period of feeding. It may be accomplished in a variety of ways. An alternate-day fast usually begins with a feast day, during which you eat as much as you like one day and then fast the next. A single 24-hour quick can be accomplished once a week, once a month, or anytime you like on a less structured schedule. You may miss a meal on a scheduled or unscheduled basis.

The approach that I recommend is the simplified eating window. It entails cramming the whole day's worth of food into a specific amount of hours. For instance, I'll eat from seven o'clock in the morning until three o'clock in the afternoon. Then easy before 7 a.m. the next day. My body would have a sixteen-hour break from digestion as a result of this. And it occurs very normally, without much thought, on occasion.

When people hear the word "fasting," they sometimes think of "starvation." People get jittery because they don't eat every few hours. What would happen if their metabolisms stopped working? Willn't they all perish at the same time? And, if they resume feeding, everything will be processed as fat, correct?

It's not about punishing yourself while you practice

intermittent fasting. It's as simple as going without food for a brief amount of time and then returning to the daily routine. Eating like a rabbit all of the time is a surefire way to manipulate your diet and lose weight. It's possible to boost your weight loss efforts and achieve your targets by eating like a rabbit for most of the day and maintaining balance and power.

In brief, none of the above issues should be a major concern. If a person is stable, that is, there is no underlying medical disorder or illness, such as diabetes, missing a meal or two may be a useful contribution to a healthy lifestyle.

About every diet book you'll find in a bookstore employs some kind of trick to get the reader to eat less. Calorie counting is time-consuming and can be frustrating. Reading labels and weighing ingredients will easily detract from the pleasure of meal preparation. Following a recipe can be daunting enough, but having to make substitutions or give up whole portions of a meal to stay within a calorie budget is not what most people want to do. Such actions also result in the diet being abandoned entirely.

An intermittent fasting strategy is a more successful way to reduce weight or retain weight. There are a few different approaches to this. Brad Pilon of Eat Stop Eat fame recommends going without eating for a full twenty-four hours. It is not a poor strategy because you'll drastically cut your calorie intake as long as you don't overdo it. The disadvantage is that living without food for a whole day is a psychological challenge that certain people would struggle to overcome.

Others recommend cramming their whole day's worth of calories into a four- to the nine-hour timeframe. This, too, is contingent on calorie counting and sticking to the diet. It's a good idea to prepare your meals some days ahead of time to not have to think about what to eat when it's time to eat. Simply cook the meals that have been prepared and go about your day.

While all of these techniques are fine and serve their functions well, a more relaxed approach will also be a successful starting point. Many people will be perfectly content to miss breakfast, have lunch later, and have a small first dinner. During the fasted time, drinking lots of water will help to stave off hunger.

If you skip a meal or two-three to five times per

week, you can lose between 1500 and 2500 calories, based on the size of the meals you're eating. When you add that all up, you're looking at about a pound of net calorie loss per week. A bigger shortfall can be problematic because it would take you longer to achieve your objectives. On the other hand, a bigger deficit is easier to handle. The ideal diet is one that you can maintain.

Finally, whether you want to miss a whole day's worth of meals, one meal at a time, or count the calories and fit them into an "eating slot," it doesn't matter. The calorie drop that results in would aid weight loss and increase your health and well-being.

Do Not Go Yet; One Last Thing To Do

If you enjoyed this book or found it useful, I'd be very grateful if you'd post a short review on Amazon. Your support does make a difference, and I read all the reviews personally so I can get your feedback and make this book even better.

Thanks

www.ingramcontent.com/pod-product-compliance
Lightning Source LLC
Chambersburg PA
CBHW070628220526
45466CB00001B/121